Most Commons in Ophthalmology
1st edition, February 2018

by
Dhaval Patel MD (AIIMS)
drdpatel87@gmail.com

This is a compilation of MOST COMMONS in OPHTHALMOLOGY.

Any contributions or comments are welcomed in the effort to improve this book. Feel free to email me at drdpatel87@gmail.com

Preface

"Most Commons" has always been the hot topic which helps in solving many direct and indirect questions in entrance examinations and also clears many fundamentals related to subject. During my ophthalmology residency at AIIMS, New Delhi, I have started gathering relevant text which has helped me to compile a huge collection of most commons and has now taken the form of this book.

Time taken to compile this book is really enormous and I have tried not to leave any topic untouched. More than 1000 ophthalmology related books has been reviewed to compile this huge list of more than 4000 "most commons". I have permitted myself to allow few duplications of most commons, it is just in the view of getting all relevant material under single heading. This Text, in a concise manner, relays information related to all major topics in ophthalmology. Additionally, it also reviews all areas commonly covered in PG and Post-PG Entrance examinations of ophthalmology.

Science is an ever changing dynamic filed and medicine is no more exception. Though each and every data collected and given here is checked for its correctness, some of the facts like percentage etc may change as new research goes on. I have taken utmost care to present the information in its latest form.

I hope readers will welcome my this text just as my previous texts like Ophthalmonics, Ophthalmology Explorer and I-Notes for which I still continue to receive appreciation emails and messages.

Dhaval Patel MD AIIMS

February 2018

TABLE OF CONTENT

Basic Sciences 9
Conjunctiva & Eyelid 27
Cornea 45
Genetics 80
Glaucoma 108
Investigations 128
Lens..146
Neuro-ophthalmology 154
Ocular Pathology 220
Ocular Pharmacology 238
Oculoplasty... 256
Oncology... 280
Optics & Refraction... 318
Refractive Surgery 332
Retina & Vitreous 343
Sclera...378
Strabismus.. 385
Surgery.. 403
Trauma & Emergencies 449
Uveitis.. 467
Miscellaneous... 503

MOST COMMONS IN OPHTHALMOLOGY

DETAILED TABLE OF CONTENTS

Basic Sciences 9
General Basics 9
Basic Anatomy 16
Basic Physiology 20
Collagen 23
Colour Vision Deficiency 24

Conjunctiva & Eye Adnexa 27
Bacterial Conjunctivitis 27
Viral Conjunctivitis 30
Allergic Conjunctivitis 32
Misc Conjunctivitis 35
Pterygium 37
Blepharitis 38
Misc Conjunctiva 40

Cornea 45
General Cornea 45
Dry Eye & Related Disorders 49
Corneal Infections 52
Corneal Dystrophies & Hereditary Diseases 62
Keratoconus & Related Disorders 67
Autoimmune Corneal Disorders 69
Corneal Graft & Keratoplasty 71

MOST COMMONS IN OPHTHALMOLOGY

Misc Cornea 77
   Genetics 80
General Genetics 80
Anterior Segment Genetics 82
Glaucoma Genetics 86
Posterior Segment Genetics 87
Misc Genetics 98
   Glaucoma 108
General Glaucoma 108
Childhood Glaucoma 115
Glaucoma Syndromes 117
Exfoliation Syndromes 121
Glaucoma Management 122
Misc Glaucoma 126
   Investigations 128
General Eye Investigations 128
Corneal Investigations 130
Corneal Topography & Tomography 131
Aberrometry 132
Glaucoma Investigations 134
Retinal Investigations 138
Orbital Investigations 142
Misc Investigations 143
   Lens & Cataract 146
General Cataract 146
Syndromic Lens Disorders 148

MOST COMMONS IN OPHTHALMOLOGY

Post Cataract Sx Complications 150
Misc Cataract 152
Neuro-ophthalmology 154
General Neuro-ophthalmology 154
Headache & Related Disorders 157
Pupil & Related Abnormalities 161
Nystagmus & Related Disorders 164
Optic Disc Related Disorders 169
Ischemic Optic Neuropathy 176
Other Optic Neuropathies 180
Brainstem Disorders 183
Internuclear Ophthalmoplegia 186
Neuromuscular Disorders 187
Intracranial Vascular Disorders 189
Facial Nerve & Related Disorders 195
Intracranial Tumors 198
Misc Neuro-ophthalmology 203
Ocular Pathology 220
General Pathology 220
Anterior Segment Pathology 221
Posterior Segment Pathology 226
Orbital Pathology 233
Ocular Pharmacology 238
General Ocular Pharmacology 238
Adverse Effects 240
Misc Ocular Pharmacology 254

MOST COMMONS IN OPHTHALMOLOGY

Oculoplasty & Orbit 256
General Oculoplasty 256
Eyelid 256
Lacrimal System 261
Orbit 265
Orbital Cellulitis 272
Thyroid Eye Disease (TED) 274
Misc Oculoplasty 277
Oncology 280
General Eye Oncology 280
Anterior Segment Oncology 281
Eyelid Oncology 285
Orbital Oncology 292
Uveal Melanoma 300
Retinoblastoma 303
Rhabdomyosarcoma 307
Neuroblastoma 308
Optic Nerve Related Tumors 309
Misc Eye Oncology 311
Optics & Refraction 318
General Optics 318
Spectacles 321
Contact Lenses 326
Computer Vision Syndrome 329
Misc Optics 330
Refractive Surgery 332

MOST COMMONS IN OPHTHALMOLOGY

Corneal Refractive Surgery 332
Lens Related Refractive Surgery 335
Complications of Refractive Surgery 336
Retina & Vitreous 343
General Retina 343
Diabetic Retinopathy 349
Age Related Macular Degeneration 352
Heriditory Retinal Disorders 353
Retinal Vascular Disorders 357
Retinal Detachments 365
Retinitis Pigmentosa 368
Endophthalmitis 369
Misc Retina 373
Sclera 378
Scleritis 378
Episcleritis 382
Misc Sclera 383
Strabismus 385
General Strabismus 385
Amblyopia 389
Esotropia 390
Exotropia 391
Fourth Nerve Palsy 392
Sixth Nerve Palsy 393
Third Nerve Palsy 394
Duane Retraction Syndrome 395

MOST COMMONS IN OPHTHALMOLOGY

Dissociated Deviation 397
Misc Strabismus 398
   Surgery **403**
General Eye Surgery... 403
Conjunctival Surgery 405
Lens, IOL & Cataract Surgery... 406
Glaucoma Surgery 418
Corneal Surgery... 425
Retina & Vitreous Surgery.. 426
Oculoplastic Surgery 434
Strabismus Surgery.. 443
Misc Surgery 446
   Trauma & Emergencies **449**
General Eye Trauma.. 449
Open & Close Globe Injury 451
Orbital Trauma 456
Chemical Injury 459
Optic Nerve Related Trauma 461
Shaken Baby Syndrome... 462
Misc Eye Trauma 463
   Uveitis... **467**
General Uveitis 467
Anterior Uveitis 469
Intermediate Uveitis... 474
Posterior Uveitis... 477
Panuveitis 485

MOST COMMONS IN OPHTHALMOLOGY

Childhood Uveitis 486
Behcet's Disease 487
Sarcoidosis 488
Syphilis 491
Lyme Disease 492
Cat Scratch Disease 493
Congenital Rubella Syndrome 494
Toxoplasmosis 495
Toxocariasis 497
Cysticercosis 499
HIV AIDS 499
CMV Retinitis 500
Misc Uveitis 501

Miscellaneous 503
Most common Race 503
Nutrition Related Disorders 504
Others 507

MOST COMMONS IN OPHTHALMOLOGY

Basic Sciences

General Basics

01. MC symptom of the eye disorders: Blurred vision

02. MC used biomedical device all over the world: Intraocular Lens (IOL)

03. MC pathophysiologic condition of the vitreous body: Posterior Vitreous Detachment

04. MC cause of superficial ocular discomfort and pain: Dry Eye

05. MC clinical test for assessing input asymmetry between the two eyes: Swinging flashlight test

06. MC optic neuropathy: Glaucoma

07. MC acute optic neuropathy in young and middle-aged adults: Optic Neuritis

08. MC pathological accompaniment of optic nerve inflammation: Demyelination

09. MC method of clinical visual field testing: Static perimetry

10. MC assessment of visual function: Measurement of visual acuity

11. MC cause of aniseikonia: Differential magnification inherent in the spectacle correction of anisometropia

12. MC form of retinopathy: Retinitis Pigmentosa

MOST COMMONS IN OPHTHALMOLOGY

13. MC species for developing genetic models of human eye disease: Mouse

14. MC cause of disseminated fungal eye infection: Candida endophthalmitis

15. MC cause of aspergillosis: Aspergillus fumigatus

16. MC manifestation of aspergillosis: Pneumonitis

17. MC mode of transmission of Aspergillus species: Inhalation of spores

18. MC used measure of visual function: Visual acuity

19. MC used instrument for measuring corneal sensitivity: Cochet-Bonnet aesthesiometer

20. MC measure of association in the literature: Odds Ratio

21. MC measurement of variability of a sample: Standard Deviation

22. MC method of sterilization:
    I. Wet steaming (autoclaving)
    II. Dry heat
    III. Aseptic filtration
    IV. ETO
    V. Irradiation

23. MC enterococci-associated nosocomial infections: Urinary tract infection followed by surgical wound infections and bacteremia

MOST COMMONS IN OPHTHALMOLOGY

24. MC molecular method used for strain characterization: Multilocus Sequence Typing (MLST)
25. MC protozoa in soil and water ecosystems: Acanthamoebae
26. MC region used in PCR to detect acanthamoeba DNA: Specific region of the 18S rRNA gene
27. MC opportunistic ocular infection: Cytomegalovirus
28. MC used solid state laser in ophthalmology: Nd:YAG (1064 nm)
29. MC form of ocular allergy: Allergic conjunctivitis
30. MC example of a microorganism with capability of producing proteolytic enzyme which can degrade the stromal ECM: Pseudomonas aeruginosa
31. MC anatomical cause of vision loss in children worldwide:
    I. Retinal Cause
    II. Corneal cause
32. MC non-Langerhans cell Histiocytosis: Juvenile xanthogranuloma (JXG)
33. MC cause of monocular diplopia:
    I. High astigmatism
    II. Changes in the crystalline lens
34. MC cause of pathological halos: Acute narrow angle glaucoma

MOST COMMONS IN OPHTHALMOLOGY

35. MC cause of dizziness: Internal ear pathologies

36. MC cause of floaters:

    I. Posterior vitreous detachment (PVD)

    II. Vitreous detachment

    III. Retinal detachment (RD)

    IV. Vitreous haemorrhage

37. MC used type of slit-lamp illumination: Parallelepiped

38. MC human ocular disorder: Myopia

39. MC measure of the central visual function: Best corrected visual acuity (BCVA)

40. MC complaint of patients with vision problems: Blurring

41. MC protozoon causing eye disease: Toxoplasmosis

42. MC used technique for antibiotic sensitivity testing: Disk diffusion test

43. MC corneal examination technique: Slit-lamp Biomicroscopy

44. MC ectoparasites of humans: Demodex folliculorum and Demodex brevis

45. MC virus known to be transmitted in utero: CMV (incidence of infection of 2.2% of all live births)

46. MC bacterial organisms found in the normal flora of the eyelids and conjunctiva:

MOST COMMONS IN OPHTHALMOLOGY

    I.   Staphylococcus epidermidis

    II.   Staphylococcus aureus

    III.   Corynebacterium species

47. MC species of Corynebacterium isolated from the human conjunctiva:

    I.   C hofmannii (Pseudodiphtheria)

    II.   C xerosis

    III.   C renale, and C mycetoides

48. MC use of photocoagulation property of laser in ophthalmology: Retinal laser

49. MC use of photoablation property of laser in ophthalmology: Excimer laser surgery

50. MC used technique for corneal photoablation: Flying-spot ablation technique

51. MC use of ionizing property of laser in ophthalmology:

    I.   Laser posterior capsulotomy

    II.   Peripheral iridotomy

    III.   laser synechiolysis

52. MC use of photochemical property of laser in ophthalmology: Photodynamic therapy (PDT)

MOST COMMONS IN OPHTHALMOLOGY

53. MC used laser delivery system in ophthalmology:
    I.   Slit lamp based laser delivery
    II. Laser Indirect Ophthalmoscope (LIO)
    III. Intraoperative Laser Endoscope

54. MC used mode for retinal laser delivery system: Continuous wave energy mode

55. MC cause of blindness worldwide:
    I. Cataract
    II. Uncorrected refractive error

56. MC cause of blindness in Western countries: Age Related Macular Degeneration (ARMD)

57. MC mode of adenoviral transmission in ophthalmology clinics: Applanation tonometry

58. MC used biopolymers in ophthalmic practice: Contact lenses

59. MC preparation used for fungal detection: KOH preparation (20%)

60. MC fluorochrome stains used for fungal detection:
    I.   Acridine orange stain
    II. Calcofluor white stain
    III. Fluorescein-conjugated lectins

61. MC site of primary infection with herpes simplex virus type 1 (HSV-1): Orofacial area served by the maxillary branch of the trigeminal ganglion

62. MC mode of transmission of HHV-8: Saliva and sexual contact

63. MC human ocular disease caused by amebas: Keratitis

64. MC illness caused by mushrooms: Mycetism (mushroom poisoning)

65. MC cause of intrauterine infection: Cytomegalo virus (CMV)

66. MC infection in first month of life: Neonatal conjunctivitis

67. MC ocular cause of photophobia: Pathologies that irritate the eye surface (traumatic abrasions, foreign bodies, herpetic and other infectious keratitis, blepharokeratoconjunctivitis, allergic keratoconjunctivitis)

68. MC light used to enhance fluorescence after the topical application of fluorescein to a corneal ulcer: Cobalt blue light

69. MC used photoscreening device for detecting amblyogenic factors in children: MTI photoscreener

70. MC used instrumentation in clinical practice to observe the anterior eye: Slit lamp biomicroscope

71. MC slit lamp method of viewing all tissues of the anterior eye: Direct Focal Illumination

MOST COMMONS IN OPHTHALMOLOGY

72. MC used slit lamp method to evaluate corneal endothelium: Specular Reflection

73. MC used device to screen patients for raised intraocular pressure: Non-contact tonometer

74. MC cause of difficulty in achieving a good retinal view while using Direct Ophthalmoscope: Being too far away from the patient

75. MC used accessory for slit lamp: Goldmann Applanation Tonometer (GAT)

76. MC principle on which most tonometer work: Corneal applanation

77. MC type of accommodative insufficiency: Presbyopia

78. MC Primary Immunodeficiency Syndromes:
    I.   IgA deficiencies
    II. Agammaglobulinemia
    III. Severe combined immunodeficiencies (SCID)

79. MC learning disability: Reading disability

80. MC form of ocular amyloidosis: Primary localised amyloidosis

Basic Anatomy

81. MC protein class in the lens: Crystallins

82. MC ganglion cell types in human retina:

    I. Midget
    II. Parasol

83. MC cells in striate cortex: Complex Cells

84. MC variation in eyelid blood supply: Lack of the peripheral arcade in the lower lid

85. MC developmental defect of the forebrain in humans: Holoprosencephaly

86. MC stromal cells in body: Fibroblasts

87. MC Descemet's membrane abnormality in ICE syndrome: Abnormal posterior collagenous layer posterior to Descemet's membrane

88. MC number of Posterior Ciliary Arteries (PCA):

    I. Two (48%)
    II. Three (39%)

89. MC type of astrocytes: Type 1B (GFAP and NCAM positive)

90. MC location of alpha and beta zone in peripapillary region:

    I.   Temporal horizontal sector
    II. Inferior temporal area
    III. Superior temporal region

MOST COMMONS IN OPHTHALMOLOGY

91. MC mesodermal brain tumor: Meningiomas

92. MC ectodermal brain tumor: Pituitary adenomas

93. MC quadrant of iris coloboma: Inferonasal

94. MC etilogical type of hypermetropia: Axial

95. MC etilogical type of myopia: Axial

96. MC corneal aging change: Corneal arcus

97. MC retinal aging change: Involutionary sclerosis of the retinal vessels

98. MC bacterium cultured from the eyelids and conjunctiva: S. epidermidis

99. MC area supplied by prepappilary loop if present:

    I. Arterial: Supplies the inferior retinal vascular system

    II. Venous: Drains the superior retinal vascular system

100. MC retinal vascular anomaly: Cilioretinal arteries

101. MC type of normal angle vessel seen in gonioscopy:

    I. radial ciliary body band vessels

    II. circular ciliary body band vessel

    III. radial iris vessel

102. MC cause of Brushfield spots:

    I. Down syndrome (80%)

    II. Normal individuals (20%)

103. MC internal position of vortex vein: 3 mm posterior to the equator

104. MC location of Clump cells of Koganei:

    I.   just anterior to the pupillary sphincter muscle

    II.   in the anterior ciliary body near the iris root

105. MC nonpigmented cell found in the choroid: Fibrocyte

106. MC location of lamina fusca: 3 to 4 mm from the limbus in the superior episclera

107. MC seen cells of conjunctival epithelium: Type II cells (with numerous electron-dense granules in the apical cytoplasm)

108. MC location of melanocytes in conjunctival epithelium: Along the basement membrane

109. MC location of giant papillae in conjunctiva: Upper tarsal conjunctiva

110. MC location of limbal girdle of Vogt: Nasal cornea

111. MC developmental abnormality of the iris: Persistent pupillary membranes (PPMs) (present in approximately 95% of newborns, and remnants are common in older children and adults)

112. MC cause of acquired heterochromia:

    I.   Fuchs heterochromic iridocyclitis is the commonest cause

    II.   Juvenile xanthogranuloma

III. Metastatic malignancy

IV. Leukemia

113. MC type of Anterior Segment Cysts: Neuroepithelial cysts (MC located at the Iridociliary junction)

Basic Physiology

114. MC leucocyte population in conjunctiva:

   I. Dendritic Langerhans cells

   II. CD68+ macrophages

115. MC symptoms of selenosis: Hair and nail brittleness and loss

116. MC deficient element causing cataract in experimental rodents: Selenium

117. MC acute response to inflammation: Hyperemia

118. MC atomic nucleus in living tissue: Hydrogen nucleus

119. MC blood-borne pathogens that we deal with in ophthalmology:

   I. Hepatitis C (Hep C)

   II. HIV

120. MC identified protein from glaucomatous Trabecular Meshwork (TM):

   Cochlin

121. MC difference in chemical composition of aqueous humour and blood plasma: Protein contents of two fluids (plasma: 6.0 to 7.0 gm/100 ml, aqueous humour: 5.0 to 15.0 mg/100 ml)

122. MC histopathologic correlate to soft drusen: Accumulation of membranous debris in basal linear deposit

123. MC presenting symptom of drusen: Decreased central visual acuity or a recent onset of metamorphopsia

124. MC peroxidized PUFAs present in Bruch's membrane of AMD: Peroxidation products of linoleic acid

125. MC polyunsaturated fatty acids (PUFA) in the retina:
    I. Arachidonic acid (AA)
    II. Docosahexanoic acid (DHA) (Highest concentration of DHA in the body is in the retina particularly in the retinal pigment epithelial cells and in the retinal photoreceptor outer segment disc membranes)

126. MC lipids in the brain:
    I. Arachidonic acid (AA)
    II. Docosahexanoic acid (DHA)

127. MC retinal glucose transporter: GLUT1

128. MC used method to produce Retinal Pigment Epithelium (RPE) from Human Embryonic Stem Cells (HESC): Spontaneous differentiation of HESC into RPE

129. MC used model to evaluate therapeutic efficacy of HESC RPE: Royal College of Surgeons rats (RCS rats)

130. MC interreceptor matrix protein in retina: Interstitial retinal binding protein (IRBP) (synthesized and secreted by rod photoreceptor cells)

131. MC form of edema in retinal vasculopathies: Vasogenic edema

132. MC Advanced glycation end products (AGE) resulting from hyperglycemia: Methylglyoxal derived AGE

133. MC used animal models of experimental diabetic retinopathy: Rats

134. MC method of diabetes induction in animal models: Streptozocin injection

135. MC method of IOP elevation in pressure induced glaucoma model of monkey: Circumferential laser photocoagulation treatment of the trabecular meshwork

136. MC form of physiological cell death: Apoptosis

137. MC visual chromophore in vertebrates: 11-cis-retinaldehyde

MOST COMMONS IN OPHTHALMOLOGY

138. MC use of PCR (Polymerase Chain Reaction) diagnostics in ophthalmology: For the confirmation of viral pathogens in cases of acute retinal necrosis

139. MC used method for detection of the PCR product: Electrophoresis in an ethidium bromide-stained agarose gel

140. MC used culture medium for M.tuberculosis: Egg-based Lowenstein-Jensen medium

141. MC technique used for the measurement of the rate of aqueous formation in the human eye: Maurice's technique

142. MC used method for assessing adaptation phenomenon: Dark adaptation or bleaching adaptation

143. MC test used for Dark Adaptation: Goldmann-Weekers adaptometer

144. MC assay used to document long term surveillance of glucose control: HbA1c

145. MC carotinoids in Lens: Lutein and zeaxanthin

146. MC connexin in outer cortical fibres of the lens: Connexin 50

Collagen
147. MC collagen molecule in the cornea: Type I (58%)

148. MC type of collagen in corneal stroma:

   I.   Type I

   II. Type V

   III. Type VI

149. MC type of collagen in Descemet's membrane: Type IV

150. MC collagen found in vitreous: Type II

151. MC collagen found in dermis:

   I.   Type I

   II. Type III

152. MC mutated gene in X-linked Alport syndrome: COL4A5 (encodes alpha 5 (V) chain of type IV collagen on chromosome Xq22.2)

153. MC dominantly inherited disorder of collagen: Stickler syndrome

154. MC cause of Osteogenesis Imperfecta: Mutation in genes encoding the alpha-1 and alpha-2 chains of type 1 collagen

Colour Vision Deficiency

155. MC cause of defective colour vision in childhood: Congenital dyschromatopsia

MOST COMMONS IN OPHTHALMOLOGY

156. MC colour vision deficiency: Anomalous trichromacy (6% of males and less than 0.4% of females)

157. MC individual type of colour vision deficiency:
    I. Deuteranomaly (reduced sensitivity to green light)
    II. Deuteranopia (complete loss of green sensitivity)
    III. Protanopia (complete loss of red sensitivity)

158. MC type of Anomalous trichromacy: Deuteranomaly (reduced sensitivity to green light)

159. MC form of red-green colour vision defects: Deutan defects

160. MC cause of deutan defect: Absence or lack of expression of the OPN1MW gene

161. MC cause of protan defect: Absence or lack of expression of the OPN1LW gene

162. MC colour deficiency in diabetic retinopathy: Tritan colour defects (due to S-cone/blue cone pathway dysfunction or S-cone cell loss)

163. MC mechanism of Inherited colour blindness: Loss or modification of Red-Green cone pigments (X linked recessive)

164. MC mechanism of acquired colour blindness: Loss or damage to blue cones

165. MC cause of cerebral achromatopsia: Infarction affecting the lingual and fusiform gyri ventral to the occipital lobe

166. MC used colour arrangement test in low vision clinics: Farnsworth Dichotomous test (the Panel D-15)

167. MC used colour vision test:
   I. Pseudoisochromatic (PIC) plate tests
   II. City University (second edition) test
   III. Farnsworth D15 and the Farnsworth-Munsell 100 hue test

168. MC used Pseudoisochromatic (PIC) plate tests:
   I. Ishihara test
   II. Hardy-Rand-Rittler test

169. MC symptom of ethambutol related optic neuropathy: Blue-yellow colour changes

170. MC type of colour vision deficiency in Dominant Optic Atrophy (DOA):
   I. Mixed colour deficit
   II. Blue–yellow colour deficit (classic but not most common)

Conjunctiva & Eye Adnexa

Bacterial Conjunctivitis

171. MC eye problem most frequently encountered by the primary care physician: Infectious conjunctivitis

172. MC infectious anterior segment disease:

    I.   Blepharitis

    II.   Conjunctivitis

    III. Keratitis

173. MC cause of conjunctivitis in children: Bacterial conjunctivitis

174. MC form of bacterial conjunctivitis: Acute mucopurulent form

175. MC pathogens causing bacterial conjunctivitis:

    I.   Staphylococcus aureus

    II.   Staphylococcus epidermidus (MC CONS)

    III. Streptococcus pneumoniae

    IV. Haemophilus aegyptius

    V.   Streptococcus viridans

    VI. Proteus

    VII. Moraxella

    VIII. Pseudomonas

MOST COMMONS IN OPHTHALMOLOGY

    IX.   Neisseria gonorrhoeae

    X.   Chlamydia

    XI.   Escherichia coli

176. MC isolated organism in chronic bacterial conjunctivitis:

    I.   S. aureus

    II.   M. lacunata

177. Mc organisms isolated from bacterial conjunctivitis in children:

    I.   Streptococcus pneumoniae

    II.   Haemophilus influenzae

178. MC gram-negative bacteria reported in chronic bacterial conjunctivitis:

    Proteus mirabilis

179. MC cause of ocular morbidity and preventable blindness in the world:

    Trachomatous chronic keratoconjunctivitis

180. MC cause of hyperacute bacterial conjunctivitis: Neisseria gonorrhoeae

181. Mc cause of infectious conjunctivitis of neonates: Neonatal inclusion conjunctivitis by Chlamydia trachomatis serotypes D-K

182. MC cause of mucopurulent conjunctivitis:

    I.   Neisseria gonorrhoeae

    II.   Neisseria meningitides

MOST COMMONS IN OPHTHALMOLOGY

183. MC coinfection with adult inclusion conjunctivitis: Gonorrhoea

184. MC etiology of the Parinaud oculoglandular syndrome: Cat scratch disease (An infectious process caused by Bartonella henselae)

185. MC agent producing phlyctenulosis: Staphylococcus aureus (In past, Mycobacterium tuberculosis)

186. MC cause of phlyctenular eye disease (PED):
    I.   Worldwide: Myobacterium tuberculosis
    II. Highly developed countries: Staphylococcus aureas

187. MC affected site in Phlyctenular Keratoconjunctivitis (PKC):
    I.   Limbus
    II. Bulbar conjunctiva
    III. Palpebral conjunctiva

188. MC sites for limbal phlyctenules: 4 o'clock and 8 o'clock positions in the inferior Circumlimbal areas

189. MC anterior segment manifestation of tuberculosis: Phlyctenular keratoconjunctivitis

190. MC bacterial cause of acute membranous conjunctivitis:
    I.   Beta-hemolytic streptococci
    II. S. aureus

III.   C. diphtheriae

191. MC cause of chronic follicular conjunctivitis: Chlamydia trachomatis (either trachoma or inclusion conjunctivitis)

192. MC type of ocular involvement with Listeria monocytogenes: Conjunctivitis

193. MC form of tuberculosis of conjunctiva:

    I.   Ulcerative form

    II.   Nodular form

    III.   Cock's comb

    IV.   Lupus form

Viral Conjunctivitis

194. MC ocular viral infection worldwide: Adenovirus

195. MC virus causing viral conjunctivitis in children: Adenovirus

196. MC cause of viral conjunctivitis:

    I.   Adenovirus

    II.   Coxsackievirus

197. MC form of ocular adenoviral infections:

I. Epidemic keratoconjunctivitis (EKC)

II. Pharyngoconjunctival fever (PCF)

198. MC cause of pharyngoconjunctival fever (PCF): Adenovirus types 3,4,7 and 14

199. MC serotypes associated with EKC (Epidemic Keratoconjunctivitis): Adenovirus 8, 19, and 37

200. MC mode of transmission of virus in EKC: Direct contact

201. MC mode of transmission of virus in PCF: Droplet spread or from contaminated swimming pools and ponds

202. MC ocular manifestation of herpes simplex virus: Blepharoconjunctivitis

203. MC ocular manifestation of congenital herpes simplex infection:

   I. Conjunctivitis

   II. Keratitis

   III. Retinitis

204. MC cause of acute membranous conjunctivitis:

   I. Adenoviral conjunctivitis caused by EKC

   II. HSV conjunctivitis

205. MC agent causing infectious mononucleosis syndrome: Epstein-Barr virus (EBV)

206. MC ocular manifestation of acquired Infectious Mononucleosis (IM): Mild self-limited follicular conjunctivitis

207. MC feature of Infectious Mononucleosis (IM): Sore throat

208. MC site of lymphadenopathy in Infectious Mononucleosis (IM): Anterior and posterior cervical lymph node chains

209. MC causes of acute haemorrhagic conjunctivitis (AHC):

    I.   Enterovirus type 70 (EV70)

    II. Coxsackievirus A type 24 variant (CA24v)

210. MC presentation of Neonatal HSV infection: Nonfollicular conjunctivitis followed by keratitis

211. MC cause of cause of the "conjunctivitis-otitis" syndrome: H. influenza

212. MC poxviral pathogen in humans: Molluscum contagiosum (previously smallpox)

Allergic Conjunctivitis

213. MC prescribed treatment of allergic conjunctivitis: Topical olopatadine hydrochloride

214. MC type of Allergic conjunctivitis:

MOST COMMONS IN OPHTHALMOLOGY

    I. Seasonal Allergic Conjunctivitis (SAC) aka Hay fever conjunctivitis

    II. Atopic Keratoconjunctivitis (AKC)

    III. Vernal Keratoconjunctivitis (VKC)

    IV. Perennial Allergic Conjunctivitis (PAC)

    V. Giant Papillary Conjunctivitis (GPC)

215. MC allergens causing allergic conjunctivitis:

    I. Various inhalant allergens, such as pollen species, Dermatophagoides pteronyssinus, Dermatophagoides farinae, various moulds (Aspergillus fumigatus, Aspergillus niger, Alternaria family, Cladosporium family, Penicillium family, Candida albicans, Thermopolyspora polyspora), animal danders (hairs, feathers, squamae), organic dusts, some foods in powder form (flour kinds, spices)

    II. Some drugs (e.g. in powder form, ointments, etc.)

    III. Digested foods

    IV. Contact allergens

216. MC aeroallergens implicated in Perennial Allergic Conjunctivitis (PAC):

    I. House dust mite (Dermatophagoides pteronyssinus)

MOST COMMONS IN OPHTHALMOLOGY

    II.   Animal dander

    III.   Feathers

217. MC type of Seasonal Allergic Conjunctivitis: Seasonal rhinoconjunctivitis (> 50% of cases)

218. MC season for vernal keratoconjunctivitis (VKC): Spring

219. MC symptom of allergic conjunctivitis: Itching

220. MC conjunctival reaction in allergy: Papillary reaction

221. MC cause of pseudogerontoxon: Vernal conjunctivitis (it takes cupid's Bow configuration) (True Gerontoxon is Arcus senilis)

222. MC location vernal shield ulcer: Upper half of the cornea

223. MC form of vernal keratoconjunctivitis (VKC):

    I.   Tarsal form

    II.   Mixed form

    III.   Limbal form

224. MC disease associated with VKC: Keratoconus

225. MC cause of Chronic Conjunctivitis: Allergy

Misc Conjunctivitis

226. MC cause of work related chemical conjunctivitis:

    I. Mepacrine

    II. Ammonia

    III. Vanadium

227. MC mode of transmission of conjunctivitis: Direct contact with secretions of sick patient

228. MC location of Ligneous conjunctivitis: Upper lid

229. MC cause of Ligneous conjunctivitis: Type 1 plasminogen deficiency

230. MC genetic cause of type I plasminogen deficiency: K19E mutation

231. Mc manifestation of plasminogen deficiency: Ligneous Conjunctivitis (to frequent exposure to ocular irritants)

232. MC genetic defect in Ligneous conjunctivitis: Lys (19) to glu mutation

233. MC cause of giant papillary conjunctivitis (GPC):

    I. Soft contact lens wear

    II. Hard contact lens wear

    III. Protruding sutures postoperatively

    IV. Use of prosthetic eyes

    V. Mechanical irritants

234. MC form of granulomatous conjunctivitis: Inflammation associated with chalazion

235. MC ocular manifestation in Pemphigus Vulgaris (PV): Purulent conjunctivitis

236. MC ocular manifestation of Erythema multiforme minor, Stevens-Johnson Syndrome and Toxic Epidermal Necrolysis (EM/SJS/TEN): Purulent or membranous conjunctivitis

237. MC inciting cause of EM/SJS/TEN:
    I. Infections (Viral MC – Herpes simplex MC)
    II. Drugs (Sulfonamides MC)
    III. Mixed

238. MC misdiagnosis of EM/SJS/TEN:
    I. Staphylococcal scalded skin syndrome
    II. Toxic shock syndrome
    III. Exfoliative dermatitis
    IV. Autoimmune bullous diseases
    V. Chemical/thermal burns

239. MC problem needing to be differentiated from the chronic phase of Stevens–Johnson syndrome: Ocular cicatricial pemphigoid

240. MC manifestation of Conjunctival GVHD (Graft Versus Host Disease): Pseudomembranous conjunctivitis

241. MC people involved in Factitious keratoconjunctivitis: Military personnel and medical field employees

242. MC symptom of Atopic conjunctivitis: Bilateral itching of the eyelids

243. MC cause of visual deterioration in Atopic Keratoconjunctivitis: Corneal complications

Pterygium

244. MC type of pterygium:
    I. Nasal (60%)
    II. Temporal (20%)
    III. Double (20%)

245. MC adjuvant therapy in pterygium surgery: Mitomycin C

246. MC cause of failure of pterygium surgery: Recurrence (0-89%)

247. MC type of astigmatism produced by pterygium: With-the-rule (steep vertical axis)

248. MC neoplasm mistaken for pterygium: Squamous cell carcinoma

249. MC cause of scleral necrosis in pterygium surgery:

   I. Mitomycin-C at a strength of more than 0.4 mg/ml or a dose of more than 0.1 cc or when applied as multiple drops over a period of weeks on to a bare sclera

   II. Beta irradiation that is too strong (more than 6000 rads)

250. MC use of limbal autografts: Pterygium surgery

Blepharitis

251. MC ophthalmic manifestations of rosacea:

   I. Meibomian gland dysfunction (manifested as SPK)

   II. Telangiectasia of the lid margin

   III. Conjunctival hyperemia

   IV. Blepharoconjunctivitis

252. MC symptoms of ocular rosacea:

   I. Foreign body sensation

   II. Pain

   III. Burning and redness

253. MC used treatment regimen for rosacea: Oral tetracyclines

254. MC associated bacteria with Bitot's spots: Corynebacterium xerosis

255. MC cause of Meibomian gland dysfunction: Obstruction of the meibomian gland orifices secondary to hyperkeratinisation of the duct epithelium or plugging with a solidified secretion

256. MC bacterial cause of blepharitis:
    I. Staphylococcus epidermidis
    II. Staphylococcus aureus
    III. Corynebacterium
    IV. Staphylococcus saprophyticus
    V. Propionibacterium acnes
    VI. Streptococcus viridans
    VII. Methicillin-resistant Staphylococcus aureus
    VIII. Budding yeast

257. MC type of blepharitis: Seborrheic meibomian gland dysfunction

258. MC cause of chronic lid inflammation: Seborrheic blepharitis

259. MC cause for trichiasis and distichiasis: Chronic inflammation of the ocular surface and eyelid (generally due to trachoma)

260. MC cause of cutaneous inflammation of the eyelid: Contact dermatitis

261. MC form of contact dermatitis of eyelid:

MOST COMMONS IN OPHTHALMOLOGY

    I.   Allergic (72%): Hypersensitivity response often related to cosmetics or topically applied agents

    II.   Irritant: Physical or chemical insult to the skin

262. MC cause of contact dermatitis affecting eyelids: Cosmetics

263. MC form of cutaneous infection of the skin of the eyelid:

    I.   Bacterial (staphylococcal)

    II.   Viral (Herpetic)

264. MC organisms isolated from patients with chronic blepharitis:

    I.   S. epidermidis

    II.   Propionibacterium acnes

    III.   Corynebacterium

    IV.   S. aureus

265. MC cause of chronic eye irritation in children: Blepharitis

Misc Conjunctiva

266. MC quadrant involved in conjunctival xerosis due to vitamin A deficiency:

Inferonasal

267. MC viral lid infection:

MOST COMMONS IN OPHTHALMOLOGY

    I.   Herpes simplex infection

    II.   Varicella-zoster infection

    III.   Molluscum contagiosum

    IV.   Papillomavirus

268. MC type of therapy used for Molluscum contagiosum: Destructive therapies like cryotherapy, curettage, topical application of keratolytics or vesicants, pulsed dye laser, and photodynamic therapy

269. MC organism seen in Malacoplakia: E.coli

270. MC age related change in eye: Conjunctivochalasis (CCh)

271. MC underdiagnosed and misdiagnosed ocular surface diseases: Conjunctivochalasis (CCh)

272. Mc location of Conjunctivochalasis (CCh):

    I.   Nasal and temporal regions of inferior conjunctiva

    II.   Middle zone of inferior conjunctiva

    III.   Superior conjunctiva

273. MC surgical management of conjunctivochalasis: Crescent excision of the affected area 5 mm posterior to the limbus

274. MC location of conjunctivochalasis: Between the eyeball and the lower eyelid

275. MC ocular finding in EDS: Epicanthal folds

276. MC ocular finding in Lyme disease: Conjunctivitis

277. MC cause of bilateral chronic papillary conjunctivitis:

    Blepharoconjunctivitis or Keratoconjunctivitis sicca

278. MC involved area in Mucus fishing syndrome: Nasal and inferior bulbar

    conjunctiva

279. MC cause of posterior (internal) hordeolum: Staphylococcus aureus

280. MC eye pathology caused by papilloma virus:

    I. Verrucous lesions of the eyelids (verruca vulgaris)

    II. Papillomas of the conjunctiva

281. MC condition of the intraepithelial conjunctival melanocyte: Benign

    Epithelial Melanosis

282. MC proliferative condition of the conjunctival melanocyte: Circumscribed

    Nevus

283. MC pigmented lesions of the conjunctiva: Benign melanocytic nevi

284. MC type of leukocyte found in conjunctiva:

    I. T cells

    II. Macrophages

285. MC OSD (Ocular Surface Disease) Challenges:

MOST COMMONS IN OPHTHALMOLOGY

    I.   DED (Dry Eye Disease)

    II.   Blepharitis

286. MC ocular manifestations of Ectodactyly–Ectodermal Dysplasia-Cleft Lip (EEC) Syndrome:

    I.   Partial or complete absence of the meibomian glands

    II.   Abnormalities of the lacrimal drainage system with resulting keratopathy

287. MC ocular disturbance in Degos' disease or malignant atrophic papulosis: Infarction of the bulbar conjunctiva

288. MC ophthalmic complication of psoriasis:

    I.   Conjunctivitis (up to 20%)

    II.   Uveitis (7%)

289. MC site for apocrine cysts of Moll: Close to the eyelashes

290. MC site of Pilar cyst/ sebaceous cyst:

    I.   Meibomian glands of the upper tarsus from retention of Meibomian gland material

    II.   Zeis glands near the eyelid margin

291. MC ocular manifestation of patients with dermatomyositis: Heliotrope rash affecting the eyelids

292. MC inflammatory myopathy of childhood: Dermatomyositis

293. MC type of Ankyloblepharon: External ankyloblepharon (lids are fused at the outer canthus)

294. MC ocular finding during acute phase of Kawasaki disease:
    I. Conjunctivitis
    II. Anterior uveitis

295. MC location of conjunctival nevus:
    I. Bulbar conjunctiva (nasal > temporal)
    II. Caruncle
    III. Plica semilunaris

Cornea

General Cornea

296. MC form of solid tissue transplantation: Corneal transplantation

297. MC form of injury to corneal epithelium: Mechanical (brought about by shear forces, blunt trauma, or laceration)

298. MC conditions associated with Filamentary Keratitis:

   I. Aqueous-deficient dry eye syndrome (KCS)

   II. Nonautoimmune and autoimmune Sjögren syndrome

   III. Superior limbic keratitis

   IV. Ocular cicatricial pemphigoid

   V. Corneal edema

299. MC causes of corneal anaesthesia:

   I. Viral infection (herpes simplex and herpes zoster keratoconjunctivitis)

   II. Chemical burns

   III. Physical injuries

   IV. Corneal surgery

300. MC cause of corneal anaesthesia in children: Congenital aplasia of the trigeminal nerve

301. MC nonspecific pathologic processes that opacify the stroma:
    I. Fibrosis (scarring)
    II. Vascularization

302. MC cause of stromal edema: Disruption of the endothelium due to
    I. The trauma of intraocular surgery
    II. As part of Fuchs' endothelial dystrophy or the ice syndrome
    III. Cases of severe iridocyclitis, herpes simplex disciform keratitis, and acute angle-closure glaucoma
    IV. Defect in Descemet's membrane and the endothelium is absent in that location either acutely (e.g. Hydrops in keratoconus, forceps injury during birth) or congenitally (e.g. Peters' anomaly)

303. MC lipid deposition in the cornea: Corneal Arcus

304. MC material deposited in Descemet's membrane: Lipid as part of a corneal arcus

305. MC cause of premature corneal arcus: Hyperlipoproteinemia types IIa and IIb

306. MC corneal opacity: Arcus senilis (Gerantoxon)

MOST COMMONS IN OPHTHALMOLOGY

307. MC source of deposits (Historically) in Descemet's membrane: Prolonged topical administration of silver-containing medications (e.g. Argyrol)

308. MC deposit in Descemet's membrane resulting from a systemic disease: Copper (which appears as the Kayser-Fleischer ring in Wilson's disease)

309. MC intraepithelial deposit: Iron line where hemosiderin pigment is deposited in lysosomes of the basal epithelial cells

310. MC iron line seen in cornea: Hudson-Stähli line (spontaneous senile corneal line)

311. MC used dye for staining ocular surface:
    I. Fluorescein
    II. Rose Bengal (rb)
    III. Lissamine green (lg)

312. MC applications of clinical confocal microscopy:
    I. Assessment of wound healing following refractive surgery
    II. Diagnosis of corneal infections

313. MC used storage medium in Europe: Organ culture

314. MC finding in acoustic neuroma:
    I. Decreased hearing

II. Corneal hypoesthesia

315. MC symptoms of corneal abrasion:

   I. Pain

   II. Photophobia

   III. Foreign body sensation

   IV. Tearing

316. MC types of human UVR (Ultra Violet Rays) injury:

   I. Welder's keratitis

   II. Snow blindness

   III. Keratitis after exposure to tanning sun lamps

317. MC cause of Superior Limbic Keratoconjunctivitis: Thyroid disease

318. MC cause of neovascularization from hypoxic injury to the cornea: Contact lens wear

319. MC used morphological technique for monitoring effective corneal preservation: Specular microscopy

320. MC cause of secondary lipid keratopathy: Herpetic keratitis

321. MC cause of delayed epithelial healing: Drug toxicity

322. MC cause of dendritic lesion in cornea: Healing abrasion

323. MC cause of secondary lipid degeneration (keratopathy): Herpes keratitis

324. MC used parameter to measure index of asphericity of cornea: Factor "Q" ($= p - 1 = -e^2$)

325. MC cause of corneal angiogenesis:

    I.   Inflammatory: Keratitis

    II.   Hypoxic: Contact lens wear

    III.   Limbal antiangiogenic barrier defect: Aniridia, chemical burns

Dry Eye & Related Disorders

326. MC long-term sequelae in patients with TEN: Dry eye

327. MC cause of Dry Eye: Age related idiopathic aqueous deficiency

328. MC ocular complication of chronic GVHD: Dry eye

329. MC involved glands in Sjogren's syndrome: The lacrimal and salivary glands

330. MC valuable examination techniques in assessing dry eye:

    I.   Ocular surface staining grading with fluorescein

    II.   Fluorescein break-up time (TBUT)

    III.   Schirmer's test

    IV.   Meibomian examination

MOST COMMONS IN OPHTHALMOLOGY

331. MC cause of delayed clearance of fluorescein dye in Fluorescein Clearance Test:
    I. Aqueous tear deficiency
    II. Meibomian gland disease

332. MC used technique for measuring tear secretion: Schirmer's test

333. MC cause of shortened TBUT: Meibum deficiency

334. MC ocular disorder associated with rheumatoid arthritis:
    I. Keratoconjunctivitis sicca (Secondary Sjogren's Syndrome)
    II. Scleritis

335. MC finding in KCS: Punctate corneal epitheliopathy

336. MC cause of evaporative dry eye: Meibomian gland dysfunction or posterior blepharitis

337. MC cause of eye drop associated dry eye: Benzalkonium chloride (BAC) which causes surface epithelial cell damage and punctate epithelial keratitis, which interferes with surface wettability

338. Mc method of treating Dry eye:
    I. Medical therapy
    II. Blockage of the lacrimal drainage system

339. MC complication of punctal plugs: Spontaneous plug extrusion (50%) (particularly common with the Freeman-style plugs)

340. MC reason for discontinuing contact lens use: Dry eyes

341. MC symptom reported by dry eye patients: Sandy, gritty feeling, soreness and scratchiness

342. MC reported severe symptom of dry eye syndrome (DES): Photophobia

343. MC used plug for temporary punctal occlusion: Freeman plugs

344. MC complication of tear-deficient dry eye: Filaments

345. MC Tear abnormality: Deficient tear volume

346. MC mode of doing permanent punctal occlusion:
    I. Disposable thermocautery
    II. Radiofrequency needle

347. MC form of dry eye: Primary acquired lacrimal disease

348. MC corneal finding of Atopic keratoconjunctivitis (AKC): Punctate epithelial keratopathy

349. MC extraocular association of AKC: Atopic Dermatitis

350. MC questionnaire used for tear abnormality screening: McMonnies questionnaire

351. MC ophthalmic complication of systemic lupus erythematosus (SLE):

    Keratoconjunctivitis sicca

352. MC lymphocyte population in Lacrimal gland:

    I. IgA plasma cells

    II. T cells

Corneal Infections

353. MC eye infection in the world: Trachoma

354. MC corneal disease: Simple corneal ulcer

355. MC cause of infectious corneal blindness:

    I. Trachoma (Developing world)

    II. Herpetic keratitis (Developed world)

356. MC cause of concretions: Late stage of Trachoma

357. MC cause of suppurative corneal ulceration: Bacterial Keratitis

358. MC risk factor for bacterial keratitis in developed countries: Contact lens wear

MOST COMMONS IN OPHTHALMOLOGY

359. MC isolate of bacterial keratitis associated with contact lens wear:

    Pseudomonas

360. MC cause of bacterial keratitis:
    I.   Staphylococcus aureus
    II. Coagulase negative Staphylococci
    III. Streptococcus pneumoniae
    IV. Streptococcus viridans

361. MC cause of bacterial keratitis in USA: Staphylococci and Pseudomonas

362. MC cause of bacterial keratitis in developing nations: Streptococci particularly Streptococcus pneumoniae

363. MC Gram-negative pathogen isolated from severe keratitis:

    Pseudomonas aeruginosa

364. MC cause of ICK (Infectious crystalline keratopathy): Alpha-hemolytic streptococci (S.viridans)

365. MC risk factor responsible for the occurrence of ICK:
    I. Prior ocular surgery
    II. Steroid use

366. MC ocular surgery predisposing to ICK: Corneal transplantation

367. MC presentation of ICK: Uninflamed corneal graft as a slowly growing, sharply demarcated, snowflake- like stromal opacity

368. MC source of recurrent HSV infection: Trigeminal ganglion

369. MC site of primary HSV infection in the facial area: Area served by maxillary division of trigeminal nerve

370. MC clinical manifestations of infectious epithelial keratitis: Dendritic and geographic ulcers

371. MC presentation of HSV keratitis: Dendritic ulcer

372. MC presentation of recurrent ocular HSV infection: Epithelial lesions (dendritic ulcer, geographic ulcer)

373. MC finding in recurrent immune stromal keratitis: Stromal infiltration

374. MC location of immune ring type of stromal infiltration secondary to HSV: Mid stroma of the central or paracentral cornea

375. MC used therapy for management of HSV stromal keratitis: Judicious use of topical steroids with prophylactic antiviral cover

376. MC presentation of endotheliitis: Disciform endotheliitis

377. MC ocular manifestation of Epstein-Barr virus (EBV) infection: Transient monocular follicular conjunctivitis

378. MC organism responsible for fungal keratitis worldwide: Aspergillus

379. MC yeast to infect the cornea: Candida albicans

380. MC serotype of Candida albicans: Serotype A (Serotype B is rare which is generally resistant to Flucytosine)

381. MC cause of fungal keratitis in India:

    I.   Aspergillus sp. (27 to 64%)

    II. Fusarium sp. (6 to 32%)

    III. Penicillium sp. (2 to 29%)

382. MC risk factors for the development of fungal keratitis:

    I.   Trauma (including contact lenses)

    II. Topical medications (corticosteroids and others)

    III. Corneal surgery (penetrating keratoplasty, LASIK, radial keratotomy)

    IV. Chronic keratitis (herpes simplex, herpes zoster, vernal/allergic conjunctivitis)

383. MC condition confused with keratomycosis: Herpes keratitis

384. MC initial stains used for the rapid identification of fungi: Gram and Giemsa stains

385. MC manifestation of human Microsporidia infection: Enteritis

386. MC ocular manifestation of microsporidia infection: Keratitis

387. MC microsporidia species causing keratitis:

    I.   Vittaforme (formerly Nosema) corneae

    II.   Encephalitozoon hellem

388. MC risk factors for microsporidia keratitis:

    I.   History of trauma

    II.   Exposure to contaminated water

389. MC appearance of Microsporidium keratitis: Coarse punctate epitheliopathy

390. MC ocular sign on herpetic keratitis: Corneal dendritic epithelial keratitis

391. MC form of recurrent HSV disease: Dendritic keratitis

392. MC cause of unilateral corneal blindness in the world: Herpes simplex viruses (HSVs)

393. MC infectious agent causing marginal keratitis: Staphylococci

394. MC location of vascular pannus in trachoma: Superior limbus

395. MC location of Herbert's pits in trachoma: Limbus

396. MC test used to diagnose oncocerciasis: Skin-snip test

397. MC diagnosed anterior eye disease in ocular oncocerciasis:

    I.   Microfilariae in the anterior chamber associated or not with iridocyclitis

MOST COMMONS IN OPHTHALMOLOGY

II. Punctate epithelial keratitis

III. Corneal microfilariae

IV. Sclerosing keratitis

V. Neovascularization of cornea leading to visual impairment and blindness

398. MC cause of mycotic keratitis:

I. Aspargillus

II. Fusarium

399. MC recovered anaerobes in Keratitis:

I. Propionibacterium

II. Peptostreptococcus

III. Clostridium

IV. Prevotella

V. Fusobacterium

400. MC dematiaceous fungus to cause corneal ulcer: Curvularia

401. MC infection in first month of life: Neonatal conjunctivitis

402. MC cause of neonatal conjunctivitis (Ophthalmia neonatorum): Chlamydia

403. MC non-infectious cause of neonatal conjunctivitis: Chemical conjunctivitis (induced by silver nitrate solution used for prophylaxis against infectious conjunctivitis)

404. MC location of corneal perforation in Gonococcal ophthalmia: Just below the centre

405. MC predisposing factor for Herpes zoster ophthalmicus: Age

406. MC involved dermatome in Herpes Zoster: T3 to L1 & Cranial Nerve V

407. MC division of trigeminal nerve affected in herpes zoster:

    I.   Ophthalmic

    II.   ature;Maxillary

    III.   Mandibular

408. MC subdivision of ophthalmic nerve affected in herpes zoster:

    I.   Frontal

    II.   Nasociliary

    III.   Lacrimal

409. MC site where varicella zoster virus (VZV) remains in latent stage:

    I.   Trigeminal ganglia (65-90%)

    II.   Thoracic ganglia (50-80%)

    III.   Geniculate ganglia (70%)

MOST COMMONS IN OPHTHALMOLOGY

410. MC areas affected by Herpes Zoster:

   I.   Thoracic dermatomes in aggregate (56%)

   II. Trigeminal nerve's dermatome (15%)

411. MC single dermatome involved by Herpes Zoster: Trigeminal nerve's dermatome

412. MC division of trigeminal nerve affected by herpes zoster: Ophthalmic division (20 times more often than are the second or third division)

413. MC division of ophthalmic nerve affected by herpes zoster: Frontal nerve

414. MC corneal presentation of HZO: Dendritic epithelial keratitis

415. MC cause of visual impairment in HZO: Keratitis

416. MC debilitating findings during the initial reactivation in herpes zoster:

   Acute neuralgia

417. MC complication of herpes zoster: Postherpetic neuralgia (PHN)

418. MC nerve palsy associated with HZO: 3rd nerve palsy (4th nerve is least affected)

419. MC indications for a surgical procedure in herpes zoster ophthalmicus: Exposure keratopathy

420. MC neurologic manifestation of herpes infection: CNS encephalitis

421. MC parasitic corneal infection: Acanthamoeba infection

422. MC species causing Acanthamoeba keratitis:

    I. Acanthamoeba castellani

    II. Acanthamoeba polyphagia

423. MC differential diagnosis of Acanthamoeba keratitis: Herpetic keratitis

424. MC predisposing condition for acanthamoeba keratitis: Contact lenses (75%)

425. MC symptom of acanthamoeba keratitis: Ocular pain (95%)

426. MC bacterial cause of Interstitial Keratitis: Syphilis

427. MC type of syphilis in which Interstitial keratitis occur: Congenital syphilis (90%)

428. MC cause of keratitis with elevated intraocular pressure: Herpes simplex virus infection

429. MC encountered cause of neurotrophic keratitis: Herpes keratitis

430. MC cause of Interstitial keratitis in developed countries: Herpes simplex

431. MC cause of unilateral Interstitial Keratitis (IK):

    I. Herpes simplex virus (71.4%)

    II. Varicella zoster virus (8.6%)

432. MC cause of bilateral Interstitial Keratitis (IK):

    I. Syphilitic IK

II. Idiopathic

433. MC systemic cause of unknown Interstitial Keratitis: Cogan's Syndrome

434. MC leprosy related threat to cornea: Lagophthalmos/corneal exposure due to Facial nerve (CN VII) damage

435. MC facial nerve divisions affected by leprous neuritis: Zygomatic and temporal leading to lagophthalmos and lower lid ectropion

436. MC external ocular infection affecting patients with HIV disease: Herpes zoster ophthalmicus

437. MC ocular finding in varicella: Vesicular eruption on the periocular skin and eyelids

438. MC used prophylaxis regimen for HSV recurrences: Acyclovir 400 mg BD

439. MC route of spread of vaccinia virus to the eye: Autoinoculation from the patient's vaccination site through contaminated fingers to his or her own face or to that of another person in close contact, that's why vaccination site should be covered until the scab detaches which can be up to 21 days

440. MC form of ocular vaccinia: Lid and conjunctival involvement

441. MC route of Entamoeba histolytica Infections: Faecal to oral transmission

442. MC clinical presentation of Entamoeba histolytica infection: Gastrointestinal infection

443. MC causes of infectious stromal melting:
    I. Developed countries: Herpes simplex virus and varicella zoster virus
    II. Developing countries: Fungal and bacterial keratitis
444. MC form of herpetic stromal disease: Immune mediated stromal keratitis (Interstitial keratitis)
445. MC form of endotheliitis: Disciform keratitis
446. MC cause of viral keratitis: Herpes simplex virus infection
447. MC predisposing factor for infectious keratitis in patients with previously healthy eyes: Contact lens wear
448. MC cause of secondary lipid keratopathy: Herpetic keratitis
449. MC lesion of onchocerciasis: Punctate keratitis with secondary fibrosis and pannus formation

Corneal Dystrophies & Hereditary Diseases
450. MC corneal dystrophy causing vision loss: Fuch's endothelial corneal dystrophy (FECD)

451. MC corneal dystrophy: Epithelial basement membrane dystrophy (EBMD) (2% of population)
452. MC encountered congenital dystrophy: Congenital Hereditary Endothelial Dystrophy (CHED)
453. MC symptom of epithelial basement membrane dystrophy: Pain associated with recurrent corneal erosion
454. MC dystrophy causing recurrent corneal erosion: Anterior basement (Cogan's or map-dot) corneal dystrophy
455. MC type of Congenital Hereditary Endothelial Dystrophy (CHED): CHED2
456. MC cause of primary recurrent erosion in general ophthalmic practice:
    I. Map-dot-fingerprint dystrophy (aka EBMD)
    II. Lattice corneal dystrophy
457. MC stromal corneal dystrophy: Lattice corneal dystrophy
458. MC cause of secondary recurrent erosion in general ophthalmic practice: Trauma
459. MC electron microscopic finding in patients with recurrent erosion syndrome: Reduplication of the basement membrane with loculated connective tissue

MOST COMMONS IN OPHTHALMOLOGY

460. MC presentation of CHED 2 (Congenital Hereditary Endothelial Dystrophy): Gray-blue, ground-glass haziness of the corneal stroma noted within the first week to 6 months of age

461. MC form of Crystalline Stromal Corneal Dystrophies: Schnyder corneal dystrophy

462. MC form of Pre-Descemet Dystrophies: Cornea farinata

463. MC clinical change in epithelial basement membrane dystrophy (EBMD): Maplike pattern

464. MC stromal dystrophy: Granular type 1

465. MC type of Macular Corneal Dystrophy (MCD): MCD type 1 (absence of antigenic keratan sulfate (aKS) from both cornea and serum)

466. MC associated corneal finding in sclerocornea: Cornea plana

467. MC form of limbal dermoid: Grade 1 (involves only corneal surface) (classification as per Mann's classification)

468. MC location of limbal dermoid: Inferotemporal limbal corneal and epibulbar region

469. MC ocular findings in Goldernhar syndrome:
   I.   Epibulbar dermoids
   II. Lipodermoids

    III.   Colobomas of the upper lids

470. MC location of dermoid in Goldenhar syndrome: Inferior temporal limbus

471. MC ocular finding in linear nevus sebaceous syndrome: Dermoid

472. MC causes of CCO (Congenital Corneal Opacity):

    I.   Anterior Segment Dysgenesis (Peters' anomaly, Sclerocornea, Dermoid, Congenital Staphyloma) : 65%

    II.   CHED: 15%

    III.   Congenital glaucoma: 15%

    IV.   Birth trauma, infection, metabolic: 5%

473. MC congenital cause of limbal stem cell deficiency:

    I.   Aniridia (incidence of between 1:64,000 and 1:96,000)

    II.   Sclerocornea

    III.   Multiple endocrine neoplasia

    IV.   Ectodermal dysplasia syndromes

474. MC corneal change in congenital aniridia: Limbal stem cell deficiency

475. MC cause of Limbal stem cell deficiency:

    I.   Chemical or thermal injuries

    II.   Ultraviolet and ionizing radiation

    III.   Stevens-Johnson's syndrome

IV. Advanced ocular cicatricial pemphigoid

V. Multiple surgeries

476. MC symptoms of limbal stem cell deficiency:

   I. Decreased vision

   II. Photophobia

   III. Tearing

   IV. Blepharospasm

   V. Recurrent pain

   VI. Redness

477. MC postoperative complications of limbal stem cell transplantation in the recipient eye:

   I. Immune rejection reaction

   II. limbal stem cell graft failure

478. MC types of choristoma affecting eye:

   I. Dermoids and dermolipomas

   II. Ectopic lacrimal gland

   III. Epibulbar osseous and neuroglial choristomas

479. MC systemic metabolic abnormality associated with corneal opacification in childhood: Mucopolysaccharidoses (except MPS-II Hunter's syndrome)

480. MC mucopolysaccharidoses: Hurler syndrome

481. MC cause of amyloidosis of the cornea: Secondary amyloidosis occurring in association with trauma (trichiasis) or prolonged inflammatory conditions

482. MC form of amyloidosis: Secondary systemic amyloidosis

483. MC presentation of primary localised amyloidosis:
    I. Lattice Corneal Dystrophy Types I (Biber-Haab-Dimmer) And III
    II. Gelatinous Droplike Dystrophy

484. MC finding in Posterior polymorphous dystrophy: Posterior corneal vesicles

Keratoconus & Related Disorders

485. MC curvatural abnormalities of the cornea:
    I. Anterior Keratoconus
    II. Keratoglobus

MOST COMMONS IN OPHTHALMOLOGY

    III.   Circumscribed Posterior Keratoconus

    IV.   Generalized Posterior Keratoconus

486. MC cause of pseudokeratoconus: Contact lens wear

487. MC ectatic corneal disorder:

    I.   Keratoconus

    II.   Iatrogenic post-LASIK ectasia

488. MC corneal dystrophy associated with typical signs and topographic evidence of keratoconus: Fuch's endothelial corneal dystrophy (FECD)

489. MC type of cones in keratoconus:

    I.   Oval cones

    II.   Nipple cones

490. MC noted slit lamp sign of keratoconus: Fleischer's ring

491. MC syndrome associated with keratoconus:

    I.   Down syndrome

    II.   Connective tissue disorders

    III.   Leber's congenital amaurosis

492. MC ocular abnormalities associated with posterior keratoconus:

    I.   Choroidal and/or Retinal Sclerosis

    II.   Lens Abnormalities

493. MC management strategy for more advance keratoconus: RGP contact lenses

Autoimmune Corneal Disorders

494. MC autoimmune disease encountered by the ophthalmologist: Corneal disease secondary to rheumatoid arthritis

495. MC collagen vascular disorder that affects the peripheral cornea: Rheumatoid arthritis

496. MC manifestation of immune mediated diseases of the cornea: Marginal keratitis

497. MC autoimmune diseases of peripheral cornea:
   I. Mooren's Ulcer
   II. PUK

498. MC disorder of the peripheral cornea: Staphylococcal marginal keratitis

499. MC collagen vascular disorder that causes PUK: Rheumatoid arthritis

500. MC cause of permanent visual loss in ocular cicatricial pemphigoid (OCP): Corneal scarring

MOST COMMONS IN OPHTHALMOLOGY

501. MC corneal abnormality occurring with rheumatoid associated scleritis: Sclerosing keratitis

502. MC cause of keratolysis: Rheumatoid-associated scleritis

503. MC condition associated with Calcific Band Keratopathy:

   I.   Hypercalcemia
   II. Chronic ocular inflammation

504. MC pattern of corneal calcification: Band keratopathy

505. MC ocular manifestation in hyperparathyroidism: Band keratopathy, a bilateral and symmetrical peripheral corneal calcification with tiny Swiss cheese-like holes and a clear interval between the band and the limbus

506. MC corneal manifestation of sarcoidosis: Calcific band keratopathy

507. MC cause of Noncalcific band keratopathy: Due to mercury preservatives (Thiomersal) in ophthalmic drops (this type of keratopathy is orange brown in colour)

508. MC ocular disease associated with band keratopathy: Juvenile Rheumatoid Arthritis (JRA, 30% to 66% of patients)

509. MC location of Band keratopathy: Interpalpebral area of cornea separated from the limbus by a clear area

510. MC age group in which Terrien's marginal corneal degeneration is seen: 20-40 years

511. MC association with Reticular degeneration of Koby: Chronic inflammation

512. MC location of thinning in Pellucid Marginal Degeneration (PMD): 4 o'clock to 8 o'clock position

513. MC ocular finding of Cogan's syndrome (nonsyphilitic interstitial keratitis, vestibuloauditory symptom and vasculitis): Bilateral peripheral subepithelial keratitis consisting of faint nummular lesions

Corneal Graft & Keratoplasty

514. MC indication of penetrating keratoplasty in paediatric age group:
    I. Developed countries: Congenital opacities
    II. Developing countries: Acquired nontraumatic scars

515. MC form of corneal graft rejection: Endothelial rejection

516. MC cause of corneal graft rejection: Allogenic rejection

517. MC associated factor with an increased risk of allograft rejection: Corneal vascularization

518. MC cause of graft failure in PK:

    I.   Graft rejection

    II.   Glaucoma

519. MC cause of late graft failure in PK: Low endothelial cell counts

520. MC postoperative complication of corneal transplantation: Astigmatism

521. MC cause of functional failure of corneal graft: Postoperative astigmatism

522. MC performed EK (Endothelial Keratoplasty): DSAEK

523. MC cause of regrafting in DSEK:

    I.   Unsatisfactory vision secondary to donor folds or wrinkles

    II.   Irregular donor lenticule thickness

    III. Interface opacities

524. MC complication of DSEK: Donor dislocation because of nonadherence of the donor against the recipient stroma

525. MC complication of DMEK: Donor graft dislocation

526. MC complication of DMAEK: Donor graft dislocation

527. MC indication for keratoprosthesis surgery:

    I.   Failed corneal transplant (55%)

    II.   Primary congenital corneal opacity (45%)

528. MC available keratoprosthetic devices:

    I.   Boston Keratoprosthesis (KPro)

II. AlphaCor™ artificial cornea

III. OOKP (osteo-odonto-keratoprosthesis)

529. MC used keratoprosthesis in US and worldwide: Boston keratoprosthesis

530. MC used keratoprosthesis in Russia: Fyodorov–Zuev keratoprosthesis

531. MC used model of the Boston keratoprosthesis: Boston keratoprosthesis type I, which is implanted in patients with intact eyelids, blink and tear film

532. MC used material for the central optical portion of the KPro: Medical-grade PMMA

533. MC postoperative complication following Boston keratoprosthesis implantation:

    I. Retroprosthetic membrane formation (25%)

    II. Elevated intraocular pressure (14.8%)

    III. Vitritis (4.9%)

    IV. Retinal detachment (3.5%)

534. MC site for initial corneal melt in Boston keratoprosthesis: PMMA/cornea interface

535. MC postoperative complication following Alphacor implantation:

    I. Stromal melting (26.4%)

II. Fibrous reclosure of the posterior lamellar opening (13.0%)

III. Intraoptic deposits (8.4%)

536. MC indication for oculoplastic intervention in Keratoprosthesis patients: Exposure keratopathy

537. MC intraoperative complication of Modified osteo-odonto-keratoprosthesis (MOOKP): Vitreous haemorrhage (0-52%)

538. MC long-term blinding complication with MOOKP: Glaucoma (7-47%)

539. MC repeat surgical procedure in MOOKP:

I. Mucosal trimming due to mucosal overgrowth at the optical cylinder

II. Mucosal grafting for extrusion of the OOKP or mucosal ulceration

540. MC methods to correct residual irregular astigmatism and refractive error after penetrating keratoplasty (PKP): Spectacles and contact lenses

541. MC performed procedure to manage high degrees of regular astigmatism post-PK: Astigmatic keratectomy

542. MC used cut patterns in femtosecond laser assisted keratoplasty:

I. Mushroom

II. Top Hat

III. Zigzag

543. MC indication of autologous limbal transplantation in world: Unilateral ocular surface burns, due to chemical or thermal injury

544. MC organisms responsible for suture abscess formation:

   I. S. epidermidis

   II. S. pneumoniae

   III. S. aureus

545. MC presenting sign of epithelial downgrowth: Glaucoma

546. MC cause of epithelial downgrowth: Cataract extraction

547. MC signs of Epithelial downgrowth:

   I. Retrocorneal Membrane

   II. Glaucoma

   III. Corneal Edema

   IV. Positive Seidel Test

548. MC cause of Stromal ingrowth: Failed corneal transplants

549. MC complication encountered during DALK:

   I. Perforation of the Descemet Membrane (DM) during surgery (10–30% of attempted cases)

II. Inadequate depth of dissection resulting in residual stromal tissue

550. MC indication of Alphacor: Corneal graft rejection

551. MC location of postkeratoplasty angiogenesis: 6 o'clock and 12 o'clock positions

552. MC cause of graft infection:
    I. Virus (MC Herpes simplex)
    II. Bacterial (Gram positive > Gram negative)

553. MC type of graft infection: Suture infection

554. MC application of corneal femtosecond lasers: Flap creation

555. MC cause for irreversible visual loss following keratoplasty: Post-penetrating keratoplasty glaucoma

556. MC corneal graft profile in femtosecond assisted DALK: Side cut angle set at 90° angulation

557. MC factor trigging the immune response against the donor tissue in patients that underwent DALK: Neovascularization of the interface

558. MC cause of reduced visual acuity and re-transplantation in Lamellar Keratoplasty: Interface haze

559. MC surgery causing Corneal intrastromal cysts: Epikeratophakia

MOST COMMONS IN OPHTHALMOLOGY

560. MC indication of systemic immunosuppression for corneal disease:

   I.   Prevention of allograft rejection in high risk cases

   II. Treatment of destructive corneal diseases considered to have an immunological basis

561. MC used hypothermic storage solution for corneal grafts: Optisol GS (Bausch + Lomb, Irvine, CA) (Includes 2.5% chondroitin sulfate, 1% dextran, ascorbic acid, vitamin B12, adenosine triphosphate precursors, and the antibiotics gentamicin and streptomycin)

Misc Cornea

562. MC source of corneal perforation:

   I.   Infection

   II. Trauma

563. MC signs of corneal perforation:

   I.   Flat or shallow anterior chamber

   II. Positive seidel test

   III. Uveal prolapse

   IV. Hypotony

564. MC cause of neurotrophic corneal disease:
- I. Ocular cause: Herpes virus infection
- II. Systemic cause: Tumors and surgeries which may damage the trigeminal nucleus, root, ganglion or any segment of ophthalmic branch of the trigeminal nerve

565. MC location of persistent epithelial defect in neurotrophic corneal disease: Superior half cornea

566. MC drugs implicated in causing Persistant Epithelial Defects:
- I. Topical anaesthetics
- II. Topical NSAIDs
- III. Topical trifluridine, beta-blockers, carbonic anhydrase inhibitors

567. MC cause of Salzmann's Nodular Degeneration (SND):
- I. Past phlyctenular keratitis
- II. Trachoma
- III. Vernal keratitis
- IV. Keratitis sicca

568. MC ocular finding in Wilson's disease: Kayser-Fleischer's corneal ring (95% of patients)

569. MC cause of direct endothelial injury: Intraocular injury

570. MC ophthalmic manifestation of Proteus syndrome:

   I.   Strabismus

   II. Epibulbar tumor

571. MC surgical management of Exposure keratopathy: Permanent lateral and/or medial tarsorrhaphy

572. MC indication of Tarsorrhaphy: To protect the cornea from exposure caused by inadequate eyelid coverage, as may occur in thyroid eye disease or facial nerve (cranial nerve VII) dysfunctions such as Bell palsy

Genetics

General Genetics

573. MC source of genetic variation in the human genome: Single Nucleotide Polymorphism (SNP)

574. MC used DNA markers in the characterization of human chromosomal fragments: Variable number of tandem repeats (VNTR) marker

575. MC used probe to screen a genomic library:
    I.   cDNA clone
    II. Positional cloning

576. MC used tissue sample for genetic testing: Peripheral blood

577. MC indication for prenatal diagnosis:
    I.   Routine screening of the general population
    II. Advanced maternal age

578. Mc methods of prenatal screening:
    I.   Ultrasound
    II. Maternal serum biochemistry

579. MC type of DNA mutations seen in humans: Genome mutations

580. MC teratogen affecting human birth: Ethanol

581. MC used isotope for DNA sequencing: S 35

582. MC aneuploidies: Trisomies

583. MC monosomy: Turner Syndrome

584. MC ocular abnormalities in Turner syndrome: Blepharoptosis and strabismus

585. MC autosomal trisomy: Trisomy 21/ Down syndrome (Mongolism) (1 in 700 live birth)

586. MC type of mutations implicated in inherited diseases:
    I. Missense mutation
    II. Nonsense mutation
    III. Frameshift mutation
    IV. Splice-site mutation

587. MC point mutation: Change of cytosine to thymine within CpG dinucleotides

588. MC tools for studying comprehensive gene expression in a tissue: Gene expression microarrays

589. MC genetic alteration detected in human solid malignancies: Mutations in the *p53* tumor suppressor gene (chromosome 17p13.1)

590. MC eye field transcription factors (EFTF) used as a marker of the eye field: RAX

MOST COMMONS IN OPHTHALMOLOGY

Anterior Segment Genetics

591. MC mutation in Gelatinous drop-like corneal dystrophy (GDLCD) :

   Gl118Stop (found in 82.5% of Japanese GDLCD patients)

592. MC form of transmission of isolated hereditary congenital cataract:

   Autosomal dominant mode

593. MC appearance of a hereditary congenital cataract: Lamellar type

594. MC ocular malformation: Persistent Hyperplastic Primary (Hyaloid)

   Vitreous

595. MC clinical and genetic types of Associated Ectopia Lentis: Marfan's

   syndrome

596. MC cause of hereditary cause of ectopia lentis: Marfan's syndrome

597. MC cause of removal of lens in ectopia lentis: Displacement of lens in AC

598. MC type of hereditary nephritis syndrome: Alport syndrome

599. MC transmission of Alport Syndrome:

   I.   X-linked (85%)

   II. AR (10%)

   III. AD (5%)

600. MC mutated gene in X-linked Alport syndrome: COL4A5 (encodes alpha 5 (V) chain of type IV collagen on chromosome Xq22.2)

MOST COMMONS IN OPHTHALMOLOGY

601. MC ocular finding in Alport Syndrome:
    I. Bilateral anterior lenticonus
    II. Perimacular retinal flecks

602. MC retinal finding in Alport syndrome: Perimacular yellow flecks

603. MC variant of CHED (Congenital hereditary endothelial dystrophy) : AR

604. MC association with adolescent keratoconus: Franceschetti's oculodigital sign

605. MC ocular abnormality associated with infantile cataract: Microphthalmos

606. MC associated ocular malformation with microphthalmos: Coloboma

607. MC genetic marker of Behcet's disease: HLA-B51 (HLA-B5101 is MC suballele)

608. MC inheritance pattern of CGD (Chronic Granulomatous Disease): XR

609. MC type of aniridia:
    I. Familial aniridia (AD) (mutations in the PAX6)
    II. Sporadic aniridia

610. MC systemic abnormalities associated with aniridia: Abnormalities in the urinary tract

611. MC eye manifestation of Fabry disease:

I. Conjunctival vascular tortuosity and ampulliform vessel dilatations

II. Corneal verticillata (whorl-like corneal opacification)

612. MC retinal finding in Fabry disease: Increased tortuosity of the vessels

613. MC symptom in Fabry Disease: Recurrent pain in the extremities

614. MC mutation in Lattice corneal dystrophy Type 2: Single guanine to adenine transition at the 654 nucleotide on the first nucleotide of codon 187 of the gelsolin gene

615. MC approach for gene therapy: Viral delivery of the gene

616. MC Adenovirus serotype used for gene therapy vector: Serotype 2 and 5

617. MC dominantly inherited disorder of collagen: Stickler syndrome

618. MC gene mutated in stickler syndrome: COL2A1 gene

619. MC cause of vision loss in Oculo-dento-osseous dysplasia (ODOD): Glaucoma

620. MC mode of transmission of Megalocornea: X linked recessive

621. MC presentation of megalocornea: Anterior megalophthalmos

622. MC mode of transmission of Microcornea: Autosomal dominant

623. MC mode of transmission of Anterior megalophthalmos: X linked recessive

624. MC ocular signs of aniridia:

    I.   Appearance of rudimentary iris

    II. Corneal pannus

    III. Cataracts

    IV. Foveal hypoplasia

    V. Nystagmus

625. MC inheritance pattern of Infantile Nystagmus Syndrome (INS): X-linked inheritance

626. MC ocular defect in Alagille Syndrome: Posterior embryotoxon

627. MC geographic location of Pseudoexfoliation patients: Scandinavia (especially Norway and Finland)

628. MC mode of inheritance of Posterior polymorphous dystrophy (PPMD): AD

629. MC genetic abnormality seen in conjunctival MALT lymphoma: Translocation t(11;18) (q21;q21)

630. MC mode of inheritance of hereditary cataracts: AD

631. MC cause of homocystinuria: Cystathionine β-synthase deficiency

632. MC ophthalmologic feature of Chondrodysplasia punctate: Cataract

633. MC abnormalities in Lowe syndrome (Lowe oculocerebrorenal syndrome):

    I.   Cataract (bilateral)

    II. Glaucoma

634. MC ocular manifestation of Tangier Disease: Corneal clouding

635. MC systemic manifestation of Tangier Disease:

    I.   Peripheral neuropathy

    II. Lymphadenopathy

    III. Splenomegaly

    IV. Orange-yellow-discoloration of the tonsils

636. MC mode of inheritance of Peter's anomaly:

    I.   Sporadic

    II. Autosomal dominant

    III. Autosomal recessive

637. MC inheritance of isolated ectopia lentis: Autosomal dominant

Glaucoma Genetics

638. MC primary glaucoma: POAG

639. MC mutated gene of OAG:

I. myocilin (MYOC) (1q23-q24)

II. optineurin (OPTN) (10p13)

640. MC mutation in GLC1A: Glu368STOP mutation

641. MC mutation identified for familial glaucoma: GLC1I

642. MC myocilin (MYOC) gene mutation: Gln368Stop mutation

643. MC adult OAG mutation: Q368STOP mutation

644. MC OPTN gene mutation: Missense mutation Glu50Lys

645. MC used method of nonparametric linkage analysis of complex form of glaucoma: Sib pair analysis

646. MC mode of transmission of Primary Congenital Glaucoma (PCG): AR

Posterior Segment Genetics

647. MC vision defect in Stargardt disease type I:

    I. Tendency to deuteranopia

    II. Decreased central vision

648. MC inherited macular disease:

    I. Stargardt disease (1 in 10000) (AR)

    II. Best vitelliform macular dystrophy (BVMD) (AD)

649. MC inheritance of Stargardt disease: AR (95%)

650. MC genetic mutation in Stargardt disease: ABCA4

651. MC mutation in Pattern dystrophy (PD): PRPH2 mutation in RDS/peripherin gene

652. MC cause of inherited blindness: Retinitis Pigmentosa (RP) (affecting 1 in 3000 persons worldwide)

653. MC RP causative gene regardless of causation:
   I.   RPGR gene (retinitis pigmentosa GTPase regulator) (MC in XLRP)
   II. Rhodopsin (RHO) gene (MC in ADRP)
   III. USH2A gene (MC in ARRP)

654. MC mode of inheritance of RP:
   I.   Sporadic
   II. Autosomal dominant: With best prognosis (22%)
   III. Autosomal recessive (9%)
   IV. X-linked recessive: Least common group with worst prognosis

655. MC form of "isolated" Retinits Pigmentosa: AR-RP

656. MC gene mutate in XLRP:
   I. RPGR (also called RP3)
   II. RP2

657. MC gene mutated in ARRP:

    I.   Usherin (USH2A)

    II.   PDE6B

658. MC gene mutated in ADRP:

    I.   Rhodopsin (RHO) gene

    II.   RP1 gene

659. MC cause of loss of visual function in RP: Macular disease

660. MC maculopathy in RP: Atrophic maculopathy

661. MC visual field defect in RP: Concentric constriction of the field

662. MC mutation in ADRP: Pro23His mutation in rhodopsin gene (12% of all ADRP)

663. MC cause of uniocular pigmentary retinopathy (unilateral RP): Blunt trauma

664. MC cause of Pseudo RP: Congenital viral diseases (rubella, measles)

665. MC form of Leber amaurosis: Isolated Leber Congenital Amaurosis

666. MC inherited form of childhood blindness: Leber congenital amaurosis (LCA aka EOSRD: Early-onset severe retinal dystrophy)

667. MC mode of inheritance of Leber Congenital Amaurosis: AR

668. MC systemic abnormalities associated with Leber congenital amaurosis (LCA): Neurologic abnormalities

669. MC gene involved in Leber Congenital Amaurosis (LCA):

    I.   CEP290 (20%)

    II.   GUCY2D (12%)

    III.   CRB1 (10%)

670. MC clinical finding in Leber's Congenital Amaurosis: Hyperopia with sluggish pupils

671. MC refractive error in Leber's Congenital Amaurosis:

    I.   Moderate hyperopia

    II.   Mild myopia (very rare)

672. MC disease associated with RP: Usher syndrome

673. MC form of deaf-blindness: Usher syndrome

674. MC form of recessive Retinitis Pigmentosa (RP): Usher syndrome

675. MC of three types of usher syndrome:

    I.   Type 1 (profound congenital sensorineural deafness and resultant prelingual deafness or severe speech impairment, vestibular symptoms, and childhood-onset retinopathy)

II. Type 2 (Partial deafness, intact vestibular functions, and a milder form of RP)

676. MC subtype of type 2 usher syndrome: Type 2A

677. MC of the genetic subtypes of BBS (Bardet-Biedl Syndrome): BBS1

678. MC gene mutated in BBS:
   I. BBS1
   II. BBS10

679. MC systemic abnormality associated with BBS (Bardet-Biedl Syndrome): Renal abnormalities

680. MC gene associated with Zellweger syndrome: PEX1

681. MC mutation in peroxisome biogenesis disorders: PEX1 mutations

682. MC mutated gene in neonatal adrenoleukodystrophy: PEX1

683. MC mutated gene in Infantile Refsum syndrome: PEX1

684. MC mode of transmission of Familial Exudative Vitreoretinopathy (FEVR): AD

685. MC foveal abnormality in X-linked juvenile retinoschisis (XLJRS, XLRS): Cystic spoke-wheel maculopathy

686. MC type of congenital retinoschisis: XLRS (1:5000 to 1:25000)

MOST COMMONS IN OPHTHALMOLOGY

687. MC cause of juvenile macular degeneration in males: Congenital X-linked retinoschisis (XLRS)

688. MC association of angioid streaks: Pseudoxanthoma elasticum (This association is named as Gronblad-Standberg's syndrome)

689. MC retinal abnormalities in PXE:
   I. fundal sheen, primarily in the temporal macula (peau d'orange)
   II. jagged cracks radiating around and away from the optic disc (angioid streaks)

690. MC mode of inheritance of PXE: AR

691. MC mitochondrial optic neuropathy: Leber's Hereditary Optic Neuropathy (LHON)

692. MC LHON-associated mtDNA mutation: The np11778 Mutation

693. MC findings in NF-1:
   I. Skin lesions
   II. Ocular lesions

694. MC finding of Tuberous Sclerosis (Bourneville Disease) in the skin:
   I. Facial angiofibromas
   II. Hypomelanotic macular ash leaf spots

695. MC ocular lesion of Tuberous Sclerosis (TS): Retinal astrocytic hamartoma (the original "phakoma" of van der Hoeve, which is present in most cases but is easily overlooked)

696. MC location of Astrocytic Hamartoma: At optic nerve

697. MC type of Astrocytic Retinal Hamartomas in Tuberous Sclerosis:
   I. Type 1: Relatively flat, smooth-surfaced, and translucent
   II. Type 2: Raised, calcified, multinodular ("mulberry-like") tumor
   III. Type 3 (Least common): Intermediate type shows features of types 1 and 2

698. MC neurological manifestation of Tuberous Sclerosis: Seizures

699. MC ocular abnormality observed in patients with tuberous sclerosis: Retinal hamartomas

700. MC renal lesion in Tuberous Sclerosis:
   I. Benign angiomyolipomas
   II. Malignant angiomyolipomas

701. MC affected organ in patients with tuberous sclerosis:
   I. Brain
   II. Kidney

702. MC cause of morbidity in Tuberous sclerosis:

MOST COMMONS IN OPHTHALMOLOGY

    I.   CNS hamartomas (subependymal giant cell astrocytoma)

    II.   Renal involvement (renal failure, renal cell carcinoma)

703. MC ocular lesion in neurofibromatosis type 1 (NF 1):

    I.   Lisch nodules (88%) (Iris hamartomas)

    II.   Choroidal hamartomas (29%)

    III.   Enlarged corneal nerves

    IV.   Plexiform neurofibromas

    V.   Symptomatic optic nerve gliomas

704. MC ocular lesions in neurofibromatosis type 2 (NF 2):

    I.   Lens opacities (67%—mainly plaque-like posterior subcapsular or capsular, cortical, or mixed lens opacities)

    II.   Retinal hamartomas (22%)

    III.   Epiretinal membranes

705. MC retinal lesion seen with neurofibromatosis: Astrocytic hamartoma

706. MC mechanism of glaucoma in patients with neurofibromatosis: Neurofibromatous infiltration and obstruction of the aqueous drainage pathways

707. MC orthopaedic problem in patients with neurofibromatosis:

    I.   Cervical kyphoscoliosis

II. Tibial bowing

708. MC type of ocular albinism: OA1 (Nettleship-Falls type) X-linked ocular albinism

709. MC form of oculocutaneous albinism (OCA):
  I. OCA2 (50% of oculocutaneous albinism) (tyrosinase positive, chromosome 15)
  II. OCA1 (tyrosinase negative, chromosome 11)
  III. OCA3 (brown oculocutaneous albinism, chromosome 9, dysregulation of tyrosinase)

710. MC mode of inheritance of oculocutaneous albinism: AR

711. MC mutation causing MELAS: A3243G mutations

712. MC manifestation of MELAS: Neurological abnormalities

713. MC mutation associated with MERRF: A8344G encoding mitochondrial mtRNA-Lys

714. MC abnormality encountered in Aland Island Eye Disease (AIED): Night blindness

715. MC known oncogenic mutation in uveal melanoma: GNAQ gene mutation (50% of UM)

716. MC genetic defects of Kjer's dominant optic atrophy (DOA):

I. OPA1 locus (Chromosome 3q)

II. OPA4 locus (Chromosome 18q)

717. MC syndromes associated with recessive optic atrophy (ROA):

I. Wolfram's syndrome (diabetes insipidus, diabetes mellitus, optic atrophy, and deafness) linked to the WFS1 gene located on chromosome 4p58

II. Behr's syndrome (progressive encephalopathy, mental retardation, ataxia, nystagmus and pes cavus) linked to the OPA3 gene located on chromosome 19q

718. MC pattern of inheritance of CSNB (Congenital Stationary Night Blindness):

I. X-linked inheritance (Xp11)

II. Autosomal dominant

III. Autosomal recessive

719. MC reasons for presentation of CSNB (Congenital Stationary Night Blindness) childhood: Nystagmus, decreased vision, and myopia

720. MC mutation found in complete CSNB: Mutations in GRM6 or TRPM1

721. MC type of somatic mutation in retinoblastoma:

I. Point mutation

II. Small deletions

722. MC karyotypic abnormality seen in choroidal melanoma: Alterations of chromosome 3

723. MC HLA subtype associated with Birdshot chorioretinopathy (BCR): HLA-A29*02

724. MC cause of autosomal dominant central areolar choroidal dystrophy: Mutation in the peripherin/RDS gene on chromosome 6

725. MC form of Niemann-Pick disease: Type A (infantile form)

726. MC reported HLA subtypes in patients with Tubulointerstitial Nephritis And Uveitis Syndrome (TINU): HLA-A2 and HLA-A24

727. MC mode of inheritance of Rod Monochromatism (Achromatopsia): AR

728. MC mutated gene in Achromatopsia:

   I. CNGA3
   II. CNGB3

729. MC ocular finding in Norrie's disease (Andersen–Warburg syndrome): Microphthalmos

730. MC mode of inheritance of Familial Exudative Vitreoretinopathy (FEVR): AD

731. MC hereditary choroidal dystrophy: Choroideremia (X-recessive)

732. MC mutation in Muir-Torre syndrome (MTS): Mutation in hMSH2

733. MC geographic location of Eales' disease patients: India

Misc Genetics

734. MC inherited disorder of the nervous system: Charcot-Marie-Tooth disease (Hereditary sensory motor neuropathy type 6)

735. MC mutate gene in Incontinentia pigmenti: NEMO gene (Xq28)

736. MC genetic risk factor for venous thrombosis: APCR (activated protein C resistance)

737. MC mutations in congenital myasthenic syndromes:
    I. Mutations that reduce the expression or alter the kinetics of the acetylcholine receptor
    II. Mutations of the acetylcholinesterase molecule

738. MC type off mutation in Myoclonic Epilepsy and Ragged Red Fibers (MERRF): Heteroplasmic mtDNA A8344G mutation

739. MC ocular abnormalities in Mucolipidosis III:
    I. Hypermetropic astigmatism
    II. Fine stromal corneal opacities

MOST COMMONS IN OPHTHALMOLOGY

740. MC mode of inheritance of oculopharyngeal muscular dystrophy (OPMD): AD

741. MC hemoglobinopathy affecting humans: Sickle cell disease

742. MC affected race by sickle hemoglobinopathies: African race

743. MC affected race by Tay-Sachs disease: Ashkenazi Jews

744. MC chromosomal abnormality seen with Synophthalmia and Cyclopia: Trisomy 13

745. MC chromosomal aberration associated with microphthalmia or anophthalmia:

    I.   Trisomy 13

    II. Trisomy 18

746. MC chromosomal aberration found in association with PHPV: Trisomy 13

747. MC cause of Osteogenesis Imperfecta: Mutation in genes encoding the alpha-1 and alpha-2 chains of type 1 collagen

748. MC mode of inheritance of Osteogenesis Imperfecta: AD

749. MC gene mutated in Osteogenesis Imperfecta: COL1A1

750. MC type of Osteogenesis Imperfecta: Type I (Osteogenesis Imperfecta Tarda)

751. MC genetic abnormality found in Merkel cell carcinoma:

MOST COMMONS IN OPHTHALMOLOGY

    I. Deletion of the short arm of chromosome 1 (1p36)

    II. Trisomy 6

752. MC form of Tyrosinemia:

    I. Type 1 (MC with no corneal involvement)

    II. Type 2 (Less common with superficial punctate crystalline lesions, often in a dendritiform pattern may mimic HSV keratitis)

753. MC inborn error of amino acid metabolism:

    I. Phenylketonuria (PKU)

    II. Homocystinuria

754. MC form of cystinosis:

    I. Infantile nephropathic cystinosis (95%) (also most severe)

    II. Intermediate Cystinosis Or The "Late Onset" Or "Juvenile" Cystinosis

    III. Ocular Or Non-Nephropathic Adult Cystinosis

755. MC posterior segment finding in cystinosis: Retinal pigment epithelial mottling

756. MC genetic disorder of copper metabolism: Wilson's disease

MOST COMMONS IN OPHTHALMOLOGY

757. MC ophthalmologic feature of Smith-Lemli-Optiz (SLO) syndrome: Blepharoptosis

758. MC ocular feature of Basal cell nevus syndrome (Gorlin-Goltz syndrome):
    I. Basal Carcinoma Of The Lids
    II. • Strabismus

759. MC sphingolipid storage disease: GM2 gangliosidosis type I (Tay-Sachs Disease)

760. MC inborn error of metabolism: Familial hypercholesterolemia (FH)

761. MC inherited coagulation disorders:
    I. Deficiencies of factor VIII (haemophilia A)
    II. Deficiencies of factor IX (haemophilia B)

762. MC genetic predisposition to venous thrombosis:
    I. Factor V Leiden mutation
    II. Prothrombin mutation

763. MC ocular manifestations of Thrombotic Thrombocytopenia Purpura (TTP)
    I. Papilledema
    II. Extraocular Muscle Palsies
    III. Visual Field Defects

764. MC ocular manifestation of Xeroderma pigmentosum (XP): Progressive atrophy of the lower eyelid

765. MC location of ocular surface neoplasm in Xeroderma pigmentosa: Limbus

766. MC histologic type of ocular surface neoplasm in Xeroderma pigmentosa:
    I. Squamous cell carcinoma
    II. Basal cell carcinoma
    III. Melanoma

767. MC ocular finding in the nevus of Ota: Scleral pigmentation

768. MC ocular complication if patients with Ichthyosis vulgaris: Ectropion

769. MC inherited neuromuscular disease in adults: Myotonic dystrophy (DM1)

770. MC ocular abnormality in patients with Myotonic dystrophy (DM1): Cataract

771. MC adult-onset muscular dystrophy: Myotonic Dystrophy

772. MC muscular dystrophy: Duchenne's muscular dystrophy

773. MC ocular finding in Mandibulofacial dysostosis (Treacher Collins syndrome): Coloboma at the outer third of the lower eyelids

774. MC associated ocular abnormalities in PHASES syndrome:
    I. Microphthalmos

II. Increased vascularity of fundus

775. MC metabolic disorder: Glucose 6-phosphate dehydrogenase (G6PD) deficiency

776. MC eye abnormality in Rubinstein-Taybi's syndrome: Nasolacrimal duct obstruction

777. MC ocular anomaly in Amniotic Band Syndrome:
- I. Colobomas of the eyelids
- II. Corneal leukomas or acquired corneal opacities secondary to exposure

778. MC ocular manifestation of Polymyositis and dermatomyositis:
- I. Heliotrope rash affecting the eyelids
- II. Iritis
- III. Conjunctivitis

779. MC ocular manifestation of Treacher Collins syndrome: Antimongolian slant to the palpebral fissures (89%)

780. MC held theory of inheritance of strabismus: Multifactorial model by Cross and Mash

781. MC mutation in Primary Gelatinous Drop-like Dystrophy (Subepithelial Amyloidosis): Gln118X mutation (founder mutation in the Japan)

782. MC ocular abnormalities associated with Alagille syndrome:

    I.   Posterior embryotoxon (95%)

    II.   Optic disc anomalies (76%)

    III.   Diffuse fundus hypopigmentation (57%)

    IV.   Iris abnormalities (45%)

    V.   Speckling of the retinal pigment epithelium (33%)

783. MC mode of transmission of Low to moderate myopia:

    I.   Autosomal dominant

    II.   Autosomal recessive

784. MC presenting sign of Meige syndrome: Blepharospasm

785. MC karyotypic abnormality in uveal melanoma: Monosomy 3

786. MC type of coloboma in Cat-Eye Syndrome (Supernumerary Chromosome 22q): Vertical iris coloboma

787. MC mode of inheritance for Ocular motor apraxia: Autosomal Dominant

788. MC mode of inheritance of Axenfeld-Rieger syndrome: Autosomal Dominant

789. MC inactivating mutation found in OPN1MW genes: C203R (substitution of arginine for a highly conserved cysteine at position 203)

MOST COMMONS IN OPHTHALMOLOGY

790. MC genetic defect in hyperhomocystinemia: Mutation in the enzyme methylene tetrahydrofolate reductase (MTHFR) leading to elevated levels of plasma homocysteine

791. MC mutated gene in stationary night blindness (fundus albipunctatus): RDH5

792. MC recognised teratogen for Holoprosencephaly: Maternal diabetes

793. MC mutation in Batten disease: CLN3, chromosome 16p21

794. MC mutation in Autosomal Dominant form of Nystagmus: PAX6

795. MC mutation in AR Cone Rod Dystrophy: ABCA4 gene mutation

796. MC ophthalmic anomalies in Trisomy 18 (Edwards' Syndrome):

   I. Epicanthus
   II. Hypertelorism
   III. Hypoplastic supraorbital ridges

797. MC cause of pseudohypertelorism: Increased distance between the medial canthi (i.e. telecanthus)

798. MC ocular finding in Frontonasal Dysplasia (Median Face Cleft Syndrome): Strabismus

799. MC ocular finding in Hallerman–Streiff syndrome (HSS, François Dyscephalic Syndrome, Oculomandibulodyscephaly):

MOST COMMONS IN OPHTHALMOLOGY

    I.   Congenital cataracts (80-90%)

    II.   Microphthalmia (78-83%)

800. MC cause of vision loss in patients of Oculo-dento-osseous dysplasia (ODOD): Glaucoma

801. MC ophthalmic feature in Brachmann–de Lange syndrome (BDLS) (aka Cornelia de Lange syndrome CDLS): Hypertrichosis of the eyebrows and eyelashes with synophrys

802. MC systems involved by Brachmann–de Lange syndrome (BDLS):

    I.   Gastrointestinal system

    II.   Cardiac system

803. MC ophthalmic abnormality in Cockayne's syndrome: Pigmentary Retinopathy (55%)

804. MC dysmorphic form of human obesity: Prader–Willi syndrome (PWS)

805. MC ocular manifestation of Prader–Willi syndrome (PWS):

    I.   Strabismus: Esotropia

    II.   Myopia

806. MC type of Epicanthal fold associated with Blepharophimosis Syndrome (BPS): Epicanthus inversus

807. MC cause of death in Alstrom Syndrome (A syndrome of retinal degeneration combined with obesity, diabetes mellitus, and sensorineural hearing loss): Progressive chronic nephropathy with eventual renal failure

808. MC type of inheritance pattern in Progressive Cone Dystrophy (PCD): Autosomal Dominant (AD)

Glaucoma

General Glaucoma

809. MC performed clinical methods for a simple assessment of the optic disc in glaucoma diagnosis and follow-up: Vertical cup to disc ratio

810. MC used primary treatment for glaucoma: Medical therapy

811. MC risk factor associated with glaucomatous optic neuropathy (GON): Elevated IOP

812. MC type of glaucoma: Primary Open Angle Glaucoma (POAG)

813. MC cause of tumor related glaucoma: Uveal melanoma (20%)

814. MC mechanisms of glaucoma in choroidal melanoma:
    I. Iris and angle neovascularization
    II. Angle closure
    III. Haemorrhage and necrosis

815. Most common neoplasm causing childhood glaucoma: Advanced Retinoblastoma

816. MC mechanism of glaucoma in retinoblastoma: Iris neovascularization

817. MC mechanism of glaucoma in iris melanoma: Direct invasion of the trabecular meshwork by tumor tissue

818. MC cause of glaucoma associated with primary or metastatic tumors of the ciliary body: Direct invasion of the anterior chamber angle

819. MC causes of glaucoma after PKP:

    I.   Wound distortion of the trabecular meshwork

    II.   Progressive angle closure

820. MC cause of secondary glaucoma:

    I.   Complicated cataract surgery

    II.   Uveitis

    III.   Blunt trauma

821. MC type of glaucoma leading to enucleation: Secondary glaucoma

822. MC cause of glaucoma blindness: PACG

823. MC cause of bilateral glaucoma blindness: PACG

824. MC masqueraders of POAG:

    I.   Chronic silent angle closure

    II.   Occult tm inflammation (trabeculitis)

825. MC diagnostic error in glaucoma: Misinterpreting chronic angle closure as POAG

826. MC cause of primary angle closure (PAC): Pupillary block

827. MC mechanism of angle-closure glaucoma: Pupillary block glaucoma

828. MC form of angle-closure glaucoma (ACG): Chronic angle-closure glaucoma (CACG)

829. MC presentation of angle-closure glaucoma (ACG): Acute primary angle closure (APAC)

830. MC timing of day in which acute angle glaucoma is common: Evening (peripheral anterior chamber is significantly shallower in the evening than in the morning)

831. MC iatrogenic cause of Acute PACG: Use of mydriatic eye-drops for diagnostic purposes in the course of an ophthalmological examination

832. MC type of PAS (Peripheral anterior Synechiae) in PACG:
    I. Chronic cases: Narrow PAS
    II. Acute cases: Broad PAS

833. MC topographic distribution of PAS (Peripheral anterior Synechiae):
    I. Broad PAS: Superior sector
    II. Narrower PAS: No such location pattern

834. MC cause of peripheral anterior synechiae in the USA: Argon laser trabeculoplasty

835. MC location of Iris processes:
    I. Nasal

II. Inferior

836. MC feature of gonio-dysgenesis: High insertion of a flat iris root, or a wrap-around type insertion

837. MC used method to examine angle: Gonioscopy

838. MC reason for using a gonioscope: Determining the relative openness of an angle

839. MC use of Koeppe goniolens: Direct gonioscopy on operating table

840. MC goniolens used in the operating room: Swann-Jacob Autoclavable Goniolens

841. MC used indirect gonioscopy lens: Goldmann type 3-mirror or 'Universal' lens

842. MC used angle grading system:
    I. Shaffer's grading system
    II. Spaeth systems

843. MC used coupling agent for gonioscopy: Methylcellulose

844. MC angle of mirror in gonioscopy lens: $62°$ (range from 59 to 64)

845. MC visual field defects in NTG (Normal Tension Glaucoma): Superior hemifield particularly the superonasal quadrant

846. MC used quantitative methods in visual field analysis: Event and trend analyses
847. MC used pressure-dependent method for aqueous humour formation rate: Tonography
848. MC method used to measure the rate of aqueous formation: Fluorophotometry
849. MC type of diurnal variation: Maximum pressure in the morning hours and the minimum pressure late at night or early in the morning
850. MC conditions with increased pigmentation of the trabecular meshwork:
    I. Pigmentary Glaucoma (In Which The Angle Is Usually Deep)
    II. Exfoliative Syndrome
851. MC Configuration of Peripheral Iris: 'Regular' or Flat
852. MC encountered ganglion cells in the human retina: Small (parvo) cells
853. MC reason to consider a patient a glaucoma suspect: Elevated IOP on routine examination or screening
854. MC mechanism by which glucocorticoids increase IOP: Accumulation of glycosaminoglycans in the trabecular meshwork by stabilizing lysosomal membranes and inhibiting the release of catabolic enzymes
855. MC site of neuroretinal rim (NRR) thinning in glaucoma: Inferior

856. MC site of notching in NRR in glaucoma:

    I. Inferotemporal

    II. Superotemporal

857. MC type of RNFL loss in glaucoma: Diffuse RNFL loss

858. MC refractive error encountered in patients with Pigment dispersion syndrome (PDS) and pigmentary glaucoma (PG): Mild to moderate myopia (60 to 80%)

859. MC conditions causing trabeculitis:

    I. Herpetic anterior uveitis

    II. Cytomegalovirus infection

    III. Sarcoidosis

    IV. Toxoplasmosis

    V. Syphilis

    VI. Posner Schlossman syndrome

860. MC identified sign in PAC (Primary Angle Closure) which indicates that treatment is required: ITC (iridotrabecular contact)

861. MC location of ONH (Optic Nerve Head) Haemorrhage in glaucoma: Superior or inferior temporal poles

862. MC cause of a "Low Patient Reliability" warning in perimetry: Excessive fixation losses

863. MC type of glaucoma in which optic disc haemorrhage can be seen: Normal Tension Glaucoma (NTG)

864. MC cause of ocular injection with increased IOP due to elevated episcleral venous pressure (EVP): Arteriovenous fistulas

865. MC types of carotid–cavernous sinus fistulas: Traumatic fistulas

866. MC example of an obstructive mechanism of elevated episcleral venous pressure (EVP): Graves' ophthalmopathy (GO)

867. MC type of uveitis associated with angle neovascularization: Fuchs' heterochromic cyclitis (in contrast to other types of uveitic neovascularization, it does not result in synechiae or angle closure and is only of clinical significance due a tendency to cause hyphema during intraocular surgery- Amsler's sign)

868. MC stimulus size used in HFA: Goldmann III stimulus size

869. MC cause of keratitis with elevated intraocular pressure: Herpes simplex virus infection

870. MC cause of blood in schlemm canal:

I. Physiologic: During gonioscopy due to compression of the episcleral veins by the lip of the goniolens (as episcleral venous pressure exceeds IOP)

II. Pathologic: Hypotony and elevated episcleral venous pressure as in carotid-cavernous fistula or Sturge Weber syndrome

Childhood Glaucoma

871. MC of glaucoma in children: Primary congenital glaucoma (PCG) (1 in 12,000 to 18,000 and 1% to 5% of all glaucomas)

872. MC presenting sign of infantile glaucoma when it presents in the first 5 days of life: Corneal edema (80%)

873. MC iris defect associated with developmental glaucoma: Hypoplasia of the anterior iris stroma

874. MC Primary childhood glaucomas associated with ocular anomalies:

I. Aniridia

II. Peter's anomaly

875. MC form of primary congenital glaucoma: Isolated trabeculodysgenesis

876. MC site of iris insertion in isolated trabeculodysgenesis: Anterior to the spur

877. MC anomaly seen in children with CIJ (congenital, infantile or juvenile) glaucoma: Presumed Mesodermal Anomaly of the Angle (Luntz) or Trabeculodysgenesis (Hoskins)

878. MC causes of poor angle visualization in young children with glaucoma:
    I. Diffuse epithelial edema
    II. Localized stromal edema associated with breaks in Descemet's membrane

879. MC iris defect associated with developmental glaucoma: Hypoplasia of the anterior iris stroma

880. MC cause of infantile onset glaucoma in neurofibromatosis: Failure of the normal angle development

881. MC mildest abnormality of iridocorneal dysgenesis: Simple embryotoxon or marginal corneal dysplasia

882. MC cause of glaucoma after trauma in childhood: Recurrent hyphema

883. MC symptom of PCG:
    I. Hazy cornea
    II. Large eyes

884. MC type of iris insertion in PCG: Flat

885. MC cause of poor vision in a kid with Primary Congenital Glaucoma: Amblyopia (and not optic nerve damage due to high IOP)

886. MC cause of Traumatic Glaucoma in childhood: Secondary to Anterior chamber haemorrhage (Hyphema)

887. MC cause of glaucoma secondary to neoplasia in childhood: Retinoblastoma

888. MC cause of uveitis causing glaucoma in childhood: Juvenile Rheumatoid Arthritis

Glaucoma Syndromes

889. MC variant of the ICE syndrome: Chandler's syndrome

890. MC presenting feature of ICE syndrome:

   I.   Pupillary distortion (In iris nevus or essential iris atrophy type)

   II. Decreased or distorted vision usually worse in the early morning (In chandler's syndrome)

891. MC feature of chandler's syndrome: Corneal edema

892. MC accepted theory on the pathogenesis of the ICE syndrome: Fundamental defect in the corneal endothelium, whose dysfunction results in corneal edema

MOST COMMONS IN OPHTHALMOLOGY

893. MC cause of Ocular Ischemic syndrome (OIS): Carotid artery stenosis (75%)

894. MC type of Sturge Weber Syndrome:
   I. Type I: Classic facial port wine stain (CM) and intracranial leptomeningeal vascular malformation, ± ocular abnormalities
   II. Type II: Facial CM ± glaucoma, but no brain abnormalities
   III. Type III: Leptomeningeal angiomatosis without cutaneous lesions or ocular abnormalities

895. MC type of hemangioma in Sturge Weber syndrome: Cavernous hemangioma or telangiectasis of the skin of the face ("birthmark" or port wine stain)

896. MC location of cavernous hemangioma in SWS: Distribution of fifth cranial nerve

897. MC phacomatosis associated with glaucoma: Sturge Weber Syndrome (SWS)

898. MC mechanism of glaucoma in Sturge Weber syndrome: Elevated episcleral venous pressure

899. MC manifestation of SWS (Sturge Weber Syndrome):
   I. Glaucoma (30%)

II. Choroidal Hemangioma

900. MC type of choroidal angiomas seen in patients with SWS: Diffuse angiomas

901. MC site of cerebral angiomatosis in Sturge Weber Syndrome: Occipital or occipitoparietal region

902. MC kind of glaucoma seen in Marfan syndrome: Secondary angle-closure glaucomas from lens-related complications

903. MC mechanism of glaucoma in Weill-Marchesani syndrome: Pupillary block angle closure by forward displacement of a small spherical lens from loose zonules or subluxation

904. MC cause of glaucoma in Juvenile xanthogranuloma: Spontaneous haemorrhage into the anterior chamber

905. MC cause of angle-closure glaucoma in nanophthalmic eyes: Relative pupillary block due to enlarged lens

906. MC abnormality in Corneotrabeculodysgenesis: Axenfeld's anomaly (posterior embryotoxon and adherent iris tissue)

907. MC systemic abnormalities seen with Axenfeld-Rieger syndrome: Teeth and facial bones abnormalities

908. MC teeth affected in Rieger syndrome: Anterior maxillary primary and permanent central incisors

909. MC condition confused with Axenfeld-Rieger syndrome: Iridocorneal endothelial (ICE) syndrome

910. MC cause of iris (stromal) hypoplasia: Axenfeld-Rieger syndrome

911. MC cause of treatment failure in NVG: Progression of underlying disease

912. MC cause for elevation of IOP in eyes with uveitis: Inflammatory damage to the trabecular meshwork

913. MC mechanism of silicone oil induced glaucoma: Blockage of the trabecular meshwork due to emulsification of silicone oil

914. MC cause of ocular hypertension in sarcoidosis: Nodular infiltration of the trabecular meshwork

915. MC mechanism of secondary glaucoma in uveitis:
    I. Blockage of trabecula with debris
    II. Peripheral anterior synechiae
    III. Iris bombe
    IV. Trabeculitis (Posner-Schlossman syndrome)
    V. Rubeosis iridis

Exfoliation Syndromes

916. MC geographic location of Pseudoexfoliation patients: Scandinavia (especially Norway and Finland)

917. MC mechanism of glaucoma in pseudoexfoliation: Trabecular block

918. MC identifiable cause of open-angle glaucoma: Pseudoexfoliation (PEX)

919. MC form of secondary open-angle glaucoma worldwide: Pseudoexfoliation (20% to 25% of open-angle glaucoma)

920. MC location of exfoliative material in pseudoexfoliation:
    I.   Pupillary border
    II. Anterior lens capsule

921. MC recognised sign of pseudoexfoliation: 3-ring sign on the anterior lens capsule, formed by a central disc, a peripheral ring, and a clear zone that separates the two

922. MC cause of PEX patients requiring surgical intervention: Lens opacification

923. MC type of cataract in Pseudoexfoliation syndrome (PXF): Nuclear cataract

924. MC cause of zonular laxity: Pseudoexfoliation

925. MC cause of "True Exfoliation" of lens capsule: Occupational exposure to infrared irradiation

Glaucoma Management

926. MC method for setting the target IOP: To aim for a percentage drop from the baseline IOP of 30-50%

927. MC forms of laser trabeculoplasty (LTP) performed for OAG:
    I. SLT (selective laser trabeculoplasty)
    II. ALT (argon laser trabeculoplasty)

928. MC complication with LTP:
    I. Transient IOP spike
    II. Mild conjunctival injection (due to lens application)

929. MC lens used for LTP: Goldmann lens

930. MC gonioscopic laser procedures:
    I. Trabeculoplasty
    II. Iridoplasty
    III. Cyclophotocoagulation of the ciliary body

931. MC used laser for trabeculoplasty: Argon

932. MC used treatment parameters for ALT: 50 μm spot size, 0.1 sec duration and approximately 800 mW power

933. MC clinical indication for trabeculectomy: Disease progression despite maximum medical and laser therapies tolerated by the patient

934. MC error resulting in failure of Laser Iridoplasty: Spot placement in the mid-periphery of the iris rather than the extreme periphery

935. MC technique used for laser iridectomy: Chipping away technique

936. MC complication of surgical iridectomy: Late cataract formation

937. MC mechanism of acute transient post-cataract surgery glaucoma: Retained viscoelastic materials

938. MC presenting symptoms of Fuchs' heterochromic iridocyclitis (FHI): Floaters

939. MC mechanism of glaucoma in Fuchs' heterochromic iridocyclitis (FHI): Degenerative changes of trabecular meshwork

940. MC lens used for laser iridotomy:
    I. Abraham lens (modified fundus lens with a + 66 diopter planoconvex button bonded to its anterior surface)
    II. Wise lens

941. MC applied laser for iridotomy: Nd YAG

942. MC cause of late iridotomy closure: Pigment migration

943. MC used technique for performing iridotomy:

   I. Direct penetration technique: Direct penetrating burns are most commonly used (50 micron spot size, 700-1200 mW power and 0.1/0.2 second exposure)

   II. "Hump" technique: Initially a "hump" is created on the iris with contraction burn of 500 μm spot size, 200-400 mW energy and 0.5-second exposure. The hump is penetrated full thickness with 50 μm, 700-1200 mW and 0.1/0.2 second burns.

   III. "Drumhead" technique: Initially stretch burns are placed circularly around the site of iridotomy with 200 μm, 200 mW and 0.2 sec. Parameters to create taughtness of the central area (Fig. 12.1) like "drumhead". The central area is penetrated with 50 micron, 700-1200 mW and 0.1/0.2 second burns.

944. MC used drug for Mydriatic Provocative Test: Tropicamide

945. MC used cyclodestructive procedure:

   I. Transscleral diode cyclophotocoagulation (TSCP)

   II. Cyclocryotherapy (it was MC used in past)

946. MC laser used for Transscleral cyclophotocoagulation (TSCP):

I. 810 nm Diode Laser delivered via a contact probe

II. 1064 nm Nd:YAG laser, delivered either with a non-contact projected beam or with a contact probe

947. MC complication of diode Transscleral cyclophotocoagulation (TSCP): Transient mild inflammation

948. MC recognized indicator of disease worsening in glaucoma: Progression of visual field loss

949. MC used agent for management of acute angle closure glaucoma: 250 ml of mannitol 20% given rapidly (intravenous drip) dose (1-2 g/kg body wt.)

950. MC used method to induce glaucoma in rats and mice glaucoma model: Episcleral vein cauterization

951. MC indication of cyclophotocoagulation: Aphakic glaucoma

952. MC used provocative test for angle closure glaucoma: Dark room prone provocative test (DRPPT)

Misc Glaucoma

953. MC type of glaucoma after congenital cataract surgery: Open-angle glaucoma

954. MC predisposing conditions for NVG (Neovascular glaucoma):
    I. Central Retinal Vein Occlusion (CRVO)
    II. Diabetic Retinopathy
    III. Ocular Ischemic Syndrome

955. MC site where neovasularization in seen in NVG: Peripupillary iris

956. MC cause of long standing glaucoma after penetrating keratoplasty:
    I. Pre-existing wound distortion of the trabecular meshwork
    II. Chronic angle closure
    III. Steroid induced glaucoma

957. MC cause of iris neovascularization: Retinal ischemia

958. MC used agent in acute angle closure glaucoma: Miotics (Pilocarpine)

959. MC type of glaucoma affecting AIDS patients: Acute bilateral angle closure secondary to anterior uveal effusion with secondary anterior rotation of the ciliary body

960. MC cause of Ghost cell glaucoma: Vitreous haemorrhage

MOST COMMONS IN OPHTHALMOLOGY

961. MC etiologic agent in patients with septic CS thrombosis: Staphylococcus aureus

962. MC causes of severe organic visual field constriction:
    I. End-stage glaucoma
    II. Severe retinitis pigmentosa
    III. Marked post-papilledema optic atrophy

963. MC cause of failure to restore vision to an alkali-injured eye: End stage glaucoma

Investigations

General Eye Investigations

964. MC unnecessary diagnostic testing in ophthalmology: Neurological evaluation of glaucoma patients with normal IOP

965. MC used glare test: Brightness Acuity Test (BAT)

966. MC used duochrome chart today: Visual acuity chart that is projected through a split red and green filter

967. MC used test for evaluating the integrity of the central field: Amsler grid

968. MC used contrast sensitivity chart:

   I. Pelli-Robson chart

   II. CSV-1000 E

   III. Vision Contrast Test System 6500 (Vistech VCTS 6500)

   IV. Optec 6500 Vision Testing System

   V. Functional Acuity Contrast Test

   VI. Multivision Contrast Tester 8000

969. MC used colour arrangement test in low vision clinics: Farnsworth Dichotomous test (the Panel D-15)

970. MC used optotype testing chart: Snellen chart

971. MC used instrument for IOL calculations: IOL master

MOST COMMONS IN OPHTHALMOLOGY

972. MC used scleral shell for immersion ultrasound:

    I.   Hansen shell

    II.   Prager shell

973. MC cause of IOL surprise:

    I.   Error in measuring axial length

    II.   Error in keratometry

974. MC application of A scan ultrasonography in ophthalmology: Axial length measurement of the globe

975. MC cause of A-scan measurement error: Beam of sound is not aimed along the visual axis

976. MC cause of falsely short axial length in A scan: Corneal compression

977. MC cause of falsely long axial length in A scan: Failure of the instrument to identify the retinal peak correctly

978. MC cause of double peak of retinal spike in IOL Master: Light reflected from the inner limiting membrane of the retina, represented by the left-hand peak, in addition to the retinal pigment epithelium, which is the right-hand peak

979. MC application of B scan ultrasonography in ophthalmology: Evaluation of eyes with opaque media

980. MC interferometer design used for OCT: Michelson interferometer with a single beam splitter that is double-passed

Corneal Investigations

981. MC method of pachymetry: Ultrasound

982. MC used confocal microscope systems:

    I.   Tandem Scanning Confocal Microscope (TSCM)

    II. Scanning Slit Confocal Microscope (SSCM)

    III. Laser Scanning Confocal Microscope (LSCM)

983. MC used Scanning Slit Confocal Microscope (SSCM): ConfoScan 4

984. MC used Laser Scanning Confocal Microscope (LSCM): HRT III

985. MC used method for quantitative interpretation in specular microscopy: Variable Frame Analysis

986. MC method for scanning the light source across the specimen in confocal microscopy: Nipkow disk

987. MC used index for polymegathism: Coefficient of variation

988. MC cause of false endothelial cell counts: Faulty calibration of the counting grid

989. MC used instrument for optical pachymetry: Haag-Streit pachymeter

Corneal Topography & Tomography

990. MC available type of corneal topographers: Placido disc based topographer

991. MC used corneal topography map: Axial map

992. MC reference surface for viewing elevation maps: Best fit sphere

993. MC used map in topography:

    I.   Surface Elevation Map

    II.   Curvature Map

    III.   Power Map

994. MC used display for Orbscan: Quad map

995. MC observed posterior corneal elevation pattern: Island pattern

996. MC topographic pattern seen in keratoconus: Inferior steepening which is more prominent temporally

997. MC cause of alteration in corneal topography: Normal contact lens wear

998. MC topographical pattern seen post-keratoplasty:

    I.   Asymmetric bow tie

    II.   Irregular astigmatism

999. MC topographic patterns seen after astigmatic keratotomy:

I. Symmetric Bow Tie

II. Asymmetric Bow Tie

1000. MC topographic patter seen after PRK:

I. Central island

II. Decentration

1001. MC suspicious topographic findings on the anterior curvature:

I. Corneal curvature greater than 47 D

II. Asymmetry between inferior and superior curvatures (I-S), where the inferior curvature is 1.4 D greater than the superior curvature

III. Skew of steepest radial axes (SRAX) greater than 20° in corneas with astigmatism greater than 1.5 D

IV. Difference in central corneal power between fellow eyes greater than 1 D

V. Distance between the apex and the center of the cornea greater than 1 mm

Aberrometry

1002. MC types of aberrometers: Hartmann-Shack and the ray tracing models

1003. MC aberration: Lower-order aberration

1004. MC higher-order aberrations responsible for night glare, halos, and ghosting:
    I. spherical aberration
    II. coma

1005. MC used method to mathematically describe the shape of the wavefront: Zernicke polynomials

1006. MC used metric in the pupil plane for wavefront analysis: Root mean square (RMS) wavefront error

1007. MC used single metric to describe aberrations of the eye: RMS deviation of the wavefront aberration surface from a plane

1008. MC used measure of wavefront flatness: RMS wavefront error

1009. MC used mathematical system to describe wavefront: Zernike polynomials of increasing order

1010. MC aberration with vector nature: Astigmatism

1011. MC induced aberration after non-customised lasik: Coma

Glaucoma Investigations

1012. MC commercial application of confocal scanning laser ophthalmoscopy (CSLO): Heidelberg retina tomography (HRT)

1013. MC method used for IOP measurement: Goldman's Applanation Tonometry

1014. MC used disposable contact apparatus with Goldman's applanation tonometer: Tonosafe

1015. MC type of tonometers used for infants and young children:
    I.   Tono-Pen (Reichert Ophthalmic Instruments, Depew, NY)
    II. I-care (Icare Finland Oy, Helsinki, Finland)
    III. Perkins (Haag-Streit USA, Mason, OH)

1016. MC type of static perimetry used in clinical practice: Standard Automated Perimetry (SAP)

1017. MC used SAP (Standard Automated perimetry) Perimeters:
    I. Humphrey Field Analyser
    II. Octopus perimeter

1018. MC used device for manual kinetic perimetry: Goldmann perimeter

1019. MC type of perimeter design used:
    I. Bowl perimeter

II. Compact perimeter

1020. MC reasons for ordering GVF testing glaucoma patients: Patients who are unable to reliably fixate for automated perimetry

1021. MC used Scanning Laser Polarimetry (SLP) instrument in clinical practice: GDx VCC (Carl Zeiss Meditec, Inc., Dublin, CA)

1022. MC biometric parameters to characterize the angle and anterior segment on UBM:
    I. Angle-opening distance (AOD)
    II. Trabecular-iris angle (TIA)
    III. Trabecular–ciliary process distance (TCPD)
    IV. Iris thickness (ID)
    V. Angle-recess area (ARA)
    VI. Iris ciliary process distance (ICPD)
    VII. Iris-lens contact distance (ILCD)

1023. MC used parameters for quantitative analysis of the angle: Angle-opening distance (AOD)

1024. MC used technique for optic disc evaluation: Direct Ophthalmoscopy

1025. MC employed threshold determination method in static perimetry: Staircase method in which true threshold is bracketed by presentations at luminance levels brighter than and dimmer than (" bracketing") threshold

1026. MC visual graphic representation of automated visual field test results: The grayscale plot

1027. MC method of adjusting the detectability of perimetric stimuli:
   I.   Stimulus Size
   II. Stimulus Luminance

1028. MC method used in perimetry for monitoring fixation: Heijl-Krakau method

1029. MC used fixation target in automated microperimetry: Single cross

1030. MC cause of arcuate field defect: Glaucoma

1031. MC retinal causes of noncongruous altitudinal defects: Disorders of the retina such as bilateral rhegmatogenous detachments or bilateral exudative detachments as seen in Harada disease

1032. MC used algorithm in Humphrey Field Analyser: Swedish interactive threshold algorithm (SITA) Standard or SITA Fast 24-2 or 30-2 threshold strategies

1033. MC cause of isolated congruous homonymous hemianopia in the absence of other neurological signs: Occipital lobe infarct from an occlusion in the posterior cerebral artery

1034. MC visual field defect in optic nerve disease: Central scotoma

1035. MC cause of diffuse depression in visual fields: Lens opacity

1036. MC causes of centrocecal scotoma:
   I.   Toxic optic neuropathies
   II. Leber's optic atrophy
   III. Optic disc pit

1037. MC damaged area of visual field in the early stage of chronic angle-closure: Superior and inferior nasal

1038. MC visual field defect in glaucoma:
   I. Nasal step or a partial arcuate defect
   II. Bjerrum's scotoma

1039. MC visual field change noted in glaucoma: Generalized depression of the visual field

1040. MC location of visual field defects in glaucoma: Bjerrum's area (or region), which includes that portion of the arcuate region that extends from the blind spot to the median raphe, where it extends 10 to 20 degrees nasally from fixation

1041. MC manifestation of visual field progression:
   I. Deepening and/or enlargement of previous scotomas
   II. New defect
   III. Diffuse sensitivity loss

1042. MC visual field defect in Optic Disc Drusen:
   I. Nerve fiber bundle defects
   II. Generalized constriction
   III. Enlarged blind spot

1043. MC pattern of non-organic visual field defects: Tunnel vision

1044. MC error introduced in Gross Perimetry method: Failure to maintain a constant distance from the patient's eye

Retinal Investigations

1045. MC method to detect and follow macular edema: OCT

1046. MC application of OCT in retinal disease: Measurement and monitoring of the retinal thickness

1047. MC ordered ancillary ophthalmic test for understanding of many vitreoretinal conditions: Optical coherence tomography (OCT)

1048. MC used dye for fundus angiography (FA): Fluorescein sodium ($C_{20}H_{10}O_5Na_2$, MW376)

1049. MC complication of fluorescein angiography:
   I. Generalized yellowish hue to the skin and conjunctiva and orange-yellow discolouration of urine
   II. Nausea and vomiting (5%)
   III. Hives (5%)

1050. MC cause of Blocked fluorescence in angiography:
   I. Blood
   II. Abnormal materials such as lipid exudate, lipofuscin, xanthophyll pigment, or melanin

1051. MC clinical use of the mfERG: To establish that a disease has an outer retinal origin

1052. MC electrophysiologic test for evaluating the RPE: Electro-oculogram

1053. MC used electrodes in Electro-oculogram (EOG): Subminiature Ag-AgCl skin electrodes

1054. MC indication for an electro-oculogram (EOG): Best's disease

1055. MC cause of negative ERG:

   I.   X-linked CSNB

   II. X-linked juvenile retinoschisis

1056. MC electroretinogram (ERG) pattern seen in CSNB with normal fundus:

   I.   Negative ERG (Schubert- Bornschein form of CSNB): Normal scotopic a-wave and a reduced or absent scotopic b-wave

   II. Reduced amplitudes of both scotopic a- and b-waves

1057. MC number of hexagons used in mfERG array: 103

1058. MC cause of poor fluorescein photographs: Involuntary movement of the patient's head

1059. MC vitreous opacity to cause Blocked retinal vascular hypofluorescence: Haemorrhage

1060. MC form of choroidal vascular filling defect: Patchy choroidal filling

1061. MC cause of staining in fluorescence angiography: Drusen

1062. MC seen scar tissue in fluorescence angiography: Disciform scar

1063. MC quantitative parameter derived from OCT datasets: Retinal thickness (obtained by segmenting the internal limiting membrane (ILM) and a boundary representing the retinal pigment epithelium (RPE)

1064. MC used noninvasive retinal measure of ganglion cell activity: Pattern ERG

1065. MC used test for early detection of maculopathies: Pattern ERG (PERG)

1066. MC used Amsler Grid type for monitoring visual fields: Grid with black lines on a white background comprising 20 rows and 20 columns of smaller squares

1067. MC ERG abnormality observed in Kearns–Sayre syndrome: Subnormal cone and rod a- and b-wave amplitude

1068. MC utilized software strategies to acquire multiple linear scans in OCT:
  I.   "Fast macular thickness" acquisition protocol
  II. "Macular thickness" protocol

1069. MC quantitative measurements studied from both the fast macular thickness and the macular thickness acquisition protocols:
  I.   Center Point Thickness
  II. Central Subfield Mean Thickness (CSMT)

1070. MC patterns of sarcoidosis found on ICG angiography:
  I.   Hypofluorescent dark spots in the early and intermediate phases of the angiogram which either become isofluorescent or remain hypofluorescent in the late phases.

MOST COMMONS IN OPHTHALMOLOGY

II. Focal hyperfluorescent spots seen in the intermediate and late phases

III. Fuzzy choroidal vessels due to perivascular choroidal leakage in the intermediate phase

IV. Diffuse zonal hyperfluorescence representing choroidal staining in the late phase of the angiogram

1071. MC fluorescein angiographic feature in eyes with the ocular ischemic syndrome: Prolonged retinal arteriovenous transit time

1072. MC used camera for neonatal ophthalmic imaging: RetCam digital camera system (Clarity Medical Systems Inc, Pleasanton, CA)

1073. MC method to determine MPOD (Macular Pigment Optical Density): Heterochromatic Flickerphotometry (HFP)

1074. MC method used to obtain Fundus Reflectance: Scanning Laser Ophthalmoscope (SLO) with 488 and 514 nm Argon laser wavelengths

1075. MC angiographical pattern of choroidal folds due to idiopathic acquired hyperopia: Horizontal arrangement of folds

Orbital Investigations

1076. MC indications for echographic evaluation of the orbit:

MOST COMMONS IN OPHTHALMOLOGY

    I.   Proptosis

    II.   Diplopia

1077. MC indication for lacrimal probing: Epiphora

1078. MC CT scan finding in orbital metastasis:

    I.   Mass (58%) well defined contrast-enhancing intraconal mass

    II.   Bone Involvement (25%)

    III.   Muscle Involvement (9%)

    IV.   Diffuse involvement (8%)

Misc Investigations

1079. MC method used for A-scan transducer alignment: Inclusion of a fixation light within the transducer probe itself

1080. MC methodology to measure aspects of the ocular circulation:

    I.   Colour Doppler imaging (CDI)

    II.   Laser Doppler Flowmetry (LDF)

    III.   Pulsatile Ocular Blood Flow (POBF)

    IV.   Angiography

1081. MC electrophysiological measures of vision function:

    I.   Electroretinogram (ERG)

II. Visual Evoked Cortical Potential (VECP)

1082. MC stimulus used for VEP testing: Checkerboard target with a pattern that reverses every half second

1083. MC used result of VEP (Visually Evoked Potentials): Measures of the P100 latency (large positive potential that, in persons with normal vision, occurs around 100 ms after stimulus presentation, it is a measure of retinocortical latency)

1084. MC stimulus used for mfVEP: Pattern-reversal stimulation

1085. MC eye movement recording techniques:
- I. Electro-Oculogram
- II. Infrared Reflection Devices
- III. Scleral Search Coil
- IV. Video-Oculography

1086. MC exophthalmometer used in clinical practice: Hertel exophthalmometer

1087. MC methods used to record eye movements:
- I. Electro-Oculography
- II. Infrared Oculography

1088. MC used noninvasive method in evaluation of carotid artery obstruction: Duplex carotid ultrasonography

1089. MC used devices to obtain digital images in camera systems: Charged coupled device (CCD) camera

1090. MC property of laser used in retinal laser surgery: Photocoagulation

1091. MC type of magnet used for medical imaging to generate a uniform magnetic field of sufficient strength: Superconductive magnets

1092. MC used Magnetic Resonance (MR) technique: Spin-echo technique

1093. MC neuroimaging abnormalities in sarcoidosis: Meningeal and leptomeningeal enhancing lesions

1094. MC used Positron Emission Tomography tracer: 18F-fluorodeoxyglucose (^{18}F-FDG)

Lens & Cataract

General Cataract

1095. MC risk factor for cataract: Age

1096. MC way of classifying cataracts: By anatomical location of lens opacities, i.e. cortical, nuclear and posterior subcapsular

1097. MC type of age related cataract:

    I.   Nuclear cataract (MC in European derived population)

    II.   Cortical (MC in African derived population)

    III.   Posterior subcapsular

    IV.   Mixed

1098. MC type of congenital cataract: Lamellar (Zonular)

1099. MC presenting sign of congenital cataract: Leukocoria

1100. MC cause of unilateral cataract in young individuals: Trauma

1101. MC cause of unilateral cataract in children: Persistent fetal vasculature (PFV; previously called persistent hyperplastic primary vitreous)

1102. MC location of cortical cataract:

    I.   Inferonasal

    II.   Inferotemporal

1103. MC method for determination of IOL position: Scheimpflug photography

MOST COMMONS IN OPHTHALMOLOGY

1104. MC used method for cataract grading in clinical studies: LOCS III (Lens Opacities Classification System)

1105. MC posterior segment abnormality found in advanced cataracts: Retinal detachment (5%)

1106. MC cause of lens dislocation (Ectopia lentis):

   I. Trauma

   II. Pseudoexfoliation

   III. Marfan's syndrome

1107. MC cause of infantile cataracts:

   I. Secondary to genetic or metabolic diseases

   II. Intrauterine infections

   III. Trauma

1108. MC lens quadrant involved both for new cataract development and for progression of pre-existing cataract: Inferonasal lens quadrant

1109. MC type of unilateral paediatric cataracts:

   I. Persistent Hyperplastic Primary Vitreous (PHPV)

   II. Posterior Lenticonus

   III. Polar Cataracts

Syndromic Lens Disorders

1110. MC anomalies associated with aberrant lens shape:

   I.   Posterior lentiglobus/lenticonus

   II. Anterior lenticonus/globus

   III. Lens coloboma

   IV. Lens umbilication

1111. MC type of cataract in Pseudoexfoliation syndrome (PXF): Nuclear cataract

1112. MC complication of intumescent cataracts: Argentinian Flag sign

1113. MC cause of small pupil:

   I. Pseudoexfoliation syndrome

   II. IFIS (intraoperative floppy iris syndrome)

1114. MC type of posterior polar cataract (PPC): Stationary

1115. MC symptom of posterior polar cataract (PPC): Intolerance to light

1116. MC ocular features of Marfan's syndrome:

   I. Myopia

   II. Lens dislocation

1117. MC direction for lens movement in Marfan's syndrome: Superotemporal

1118. MC vertebral anomaly in Marfan's syndrome: Kyphoscoliosis

MOST COMMONS IN OPHTHALMOLOGY

1119. MC cause of death in Marfan's syndrome:

    I.   Childhood: Mitral valve disease

    II.   Adults: Dissecting aortic aneurysm

1120. MC direction for lens movement in homocystinuria: Inferonasal

1121. MC symptoms of homocystinuria:

    I.   Lens dislocation (95%)

    II.   Mental retardation (88%)

    III.   Dental abnormalities (40%)

    IV.   Arachnodactyly (13%)

1122. MC primary defect in homocystinuria: Fraying and disruption of the zonular fibers that anchor the lens to the ciliary body

1123. MC presentation of homocystinuria in paediatric population: Developmental delay

1124. MC skeletal manifestation of homocystinuria: Osteoporosis

1125. MC bone involved by osteoporosis in homocystinuria:

    I.   Spine

    II.   Long bones

1126. MC cause of death in Homocystinuria: Thromboembolism

1127. MC syndrome associated with microspherophakia: Weill-Marchesani syndrome

1128. MC presentation of Hereditary Hyperferritinemia-Cataract Syndrome (HHCS): Childhood and adolescence patients with symptoms of glare and severe photophobia that exceeds visual loss

Post Cataract Sx Complications

1129. MC cause of PCO: Fibrotic plaques

1130. MC complication of cataract surgery: Posterior capsular opacification

1131. MC used laser for treating PCO: Nd:YAG Laser

1132. MC cause of zonular laxity: Pseudoexfoliation

1133. MC symptom of TASS (Toxic Anterior Segment Syndrome): Markedly blurred vision immediately after cataract surgery

1134. MC sign of TASS: Diffuse limbus to limbus corneal edema

1135. MC cause of TASS: Inadequate cleaning of phacoemulsification and irrigation/aspiration (I/A) handpieces

1136. MC cause of Uveitis-glaucoma-hyphema (UGH), or Ellingson's syndrome:

MOST COMMONS IN OPHTHALMOLOGY

    I.   Previously: Closed-loop anterior chamber lenses

    II.   Now: Noncapsular bag fixated posterior chamber IOLs (Single piece PCIOL in sulcus)

1137. MC complication of Nd:YAG Laser Capsulotomy:

    I.   IOL pitting

    II.   Anterior Hyaloid face rupture

1138. MC time interval between Nd:YAG laser capsulotomy and onset of rhegmatogenous retinal detachment: 5 to 7 months

1139. MC reason for wearing glasses after MFIOL implantation: Preoperative astigmatism

1140. MC uveitis-related postoperative complications of cataract surgery:

    I.   Cystoid macular edema

    II.   Hypotony and synechia formation

1141. MC cause of irregular pupil after Infantile cataract surgery: Posterior synechiae between the iris and the residual lens capsule

1142. MC anterior segment vitreous strand configurations to the corneoscleral wound:

    I.   A narrow discrete vitreous strand

II. A broad sheet of vitreous without incarceration of iris at the wound

III. A medium to broadsheet of vitreous band with either tenting upwards of iris due to adhesion or incarceration of iris to the cataract wound along with the vitreous band

1143. MC complication in the small incision cataract extraction by manual phacocracking: Corneal edema

Misc Cataract

1144. MC type of cataract associated with phakic-IOLs: Anterior subcapsular cataracts

1145. MC metabolic cause of cataract development: Diabetes mellitus

1146. MC toxic agent causing cataract: Steroid

1147. MC metabolic disturbance causing cataract during infancy: Galactosemia

1148. MC type of cataract associated with Smoking: Nuclear sclerosis

1149. MC ocular sign of dyslipidemia: Cortical lenticular opacification

1150. MC systemic sign of dyslipidemia: Achilles tendon thickening

1151. MC cause of secondary cataract: Chronic anterior uveitis

MOST COMMONS IN OPHTHALMOLOGY

1152. MC eye involved in Radiation cataract: Left eye (the eye which in a right-handed worker is nearer the furnace)

1153. MC causes of Toxic Cataracts:

    I.   Ergot poisoning (usually from eating rye bread)

    II.   Naphthalene

    III.   Thallium

    IV.   Dinitrophenol, which is sometimes taken for slimming

    V.   Steroid therapy

1154. MC ocular change after Electric Shock: Cataract

Neuro-ophthalmology

General Neuro-ophthalmology

1155. MC cause of single or multiple cranial nerve palsy: Head injury

1156. MC problem faced by the neurologist in the differential diagnosis of visual loss: Deciding whether the visual loss is the result of a lesion of the optic nerve or a lesion of the macula

1157. MC ophthalmic presentation of a unilateral disc anomaly: Strabismus

1158. MC ophthalmic presentation of a bilateral disc anomalies: Poor vision or nystagmus at younger age

1159. MC form of Anisocoria: Physiologic or essential anisocoria (difference in pupil size of 0.4 mm or more)

1160. MC location for a cerebral aneurysm with third nerve palsy: Junction of PCA (posterior communicating artery) & ICA (internal carotid artery)

1161. MC circulation involved by Berry's aneurysm: Posterior vertebrobasilar system

1162. MC location of Berry's aneurysm: At the origin of the posterior communicating artery from the internal carotid artery

1163. MC cause of a bitemporal field defect: A pituitary gland tumor

1164. MC cause of acquired epilepsy worldwide: Cysticercosis

MOST COMMONS IN OPHTHALMOLOGY

1165. MC pattern of chiasmal field loss: Bitemporal hemianopia

1166. MC form of referred eye pain: Occipital neuralgia (pain is generated by the back of the neck, but sent the message to the brain that the eyes hurt)

1167. MC location of melanocytoma (type of uveal tract nevus): Optic disc (Peripapillary region)

1168. MC factor precipitating amaurosis fugax: Change in posture

1169. MC symptom of carotid artery disease: Amaurosis fugax (a type of TIA)

1170. MC clinical sign of a circulatory disorder of the optic nerve: Amaurosis fugax

1171. MC efferent neuroophthalmic complaint: Double vision

1172. MC eye movement in Bell's phenomenon: Eyes rotate up and out

1173. MC fungal infection of the CNS: Cryptococcus

1174. MC fungal cause of optic neuropathy: Cryptococcus

1175. MC cranial nerve involved in Carcinomatous meningitis:
    I. Third nerve
    II. Sixth nerve
    III. facial nerve
    IV. trigeminal nerve

V. acoustic nerve

1176. MC visual disorders in infants with poor vision, nystagmus, and a seemingly normal ocular examination:
   I. LCA (Leber's Congenital Amaurosis): Extinguished or markedly attenuated ERG
   II. CSNB (Congenital Stationary Night Blindness): Normal a wave but an attenuated b wave on rod-mediated ERG; the cone-mediated ERG may also be abnormal
   III. Congenital achromatopsia: Attenuated or nonremarkable cone-mediated ERG (rod mediated ERG is spared)

1177. MC Congenital Stationary Dark Adaptation Disorders:
   I. Congenital stationary night blindness
   II. Fundus albipunctatus
   III. Oguchi's disease

1178. MC nonorganic disturbance in ophthalmology: Decreased visual acuity

1179. MC pattern of nonorganic/functional loss of vision: Visual acuity loss with normal visual fields

1180. MC nonorganic visual field defect: Non-specifically constricted visual field

1181. MC nonorganic disturbance of ocular motility and alignment: Spasm of the near reflex

1182. MC nonorganic pupillary disturbance seen in ophthalmologic practice: Unilateral (and occasionally bilateral) fixed dilated pupil caused by topical administration of a mydriatic agent

1183. MC association with formed visual hallucinations: Temporal lobe lesion

1184. MC association with unformed visual hallucinations: Occipital lobe lesion

1185. MC lesions responsible for gaze-evoked amaurosis:
   I. Cavernous haemangiomas
   II. Optic nerve sheath meningiomas

1186. MC pattern of visual field loss in Neuroretinitis: Central or cecocentral scotoma from edema of the papillomacular bundle

Headache & Related Disorders

1187. MC cause for cooperative interaction between neurologists and ophthalmologists: Headache

1188. MC type of headache: Stress headache

1189. MC nonvisual symptom of papilledema: Headache

1190. MC symptom of patients with raised ICP: Headache

MOST COMMONS IN OPHTHALMOLOGY

1191. MC cause of intense and incapacitating headache of abrupt onset:

    Subarachnoid haemorrhage (SAH)

1192. MC symptom of pinealoma: Headache

1193. MC neurological manifestation of pituitary tumors: Headache

1194. MC type of chronic recurring pain: Tension Headache

1195. MC form of primary headache: Tension-type headache (TTH)

1196. MC type of primary headache syndromes:

    I.   Migraine
    II. Tension type headache

1197. MC cause of episodic visual loss disturbances in childhood: Migraine

1198. MC cause of unilateral dilation during a migraine attack:

    Parasympathetic hypofunction

1199. MC triggers for migraine attacks:

    I.   Stress
    II. Hormonal changes

1200. MC cause of pathologic micropsia: Migraine

1201. MC cause of migraine like headache: Medication Overuse Headache (MOH)

1202. MC type of migraine: Migraine without aura

MOST COMMONS IN OPHTHALMOLOGY

1203. MC type of visual defect in transient migraine disease:

   I. Scintillating scotoma

   II. Hemianopias

   III. Monocular visual loss

1204. MC cause of bilateral transient visual loss:

   I. Migraine visual aura

   II. Occipital transient ischemic attack

   III. Occipital seizures

1205. MC type of aura in migraine:

   I. Visual aura (Fortification scotoma)

   II. Sensory disturbance

1206. MC description of visual aura of migraine: Unilateral (binocular) geometric zigzag figure that usually begins in the center of the visual field and gradually extends to the periphery over a period of 15 to 30 min

1207. MC presentation of cerebral venous sinus thrombosis (CVT): New onset of headache with a focal neurologic deficit or a partial seizure

1208. MC clinical symptom of intracranial hypotension: Headache

1209. MC used treatment for persistent low-pressure headache: Epidural blood patch

1210. MC presentation of internal carotid artery dissection: Headache with ipsilateral ophthalmic signs and contralateral neurologic deficits

1211. MC cause of referred orbital pain: Tension headache

1212. MC ophthalmic cause of headache:
- I. Refractive error
- II. Eyestrain from convergence insufficiency
- III. Glaucoma
- IV. Dry eyes
- V. Uveitis
- VI. Optic neuritis

1213. MC cause of refractive headache: Uncorrected Hypermetropes

1214. MC type of eye related headaches:
- I. Frontal and brow-ache: Refractive error and convergence excess
- II. Occipital: Convergence insufficiency and vertical imbalance
- III. Temporal: Uncorrected oblique astigmatism

1215. MC sequela of complicated migraine: Occipital lobe infarct with a homonymous field defects

Pupil & Related Abnormalities

1216. MC method to perform Relative Afferent Pupillary Defect (RAPD) test: Swinging flashlight test (SFT)

1217. MC site of damage in an RAPD: Optic nerve

1218. MC pupillary disturbance seen in patients with MS: Relative afferent pupillary defect (RAPD)

1219. MC pupillary abnormality associated with GCA:
   I. Relative APD (RAPD)
   II. Tonic Pupil
   III. Horner's Syndrome

1220. MC causes of central LND (Light Near Dissociation):
   I. Stroke
   II. Pineal Tumors
   III. Hydrocephalus

1221. MC cause of isolated internal ophthalmoplegia: Tonic pupil

1222. MC cause of a tonic pupil: Adie (or Holmes Adie) syndrome

MOST COMMONS IN OPHTHALMOLOGY

1223. MC used pharmacologic agent for demonstrating supersensitivity in Adie's tonic pupil: Diluted (1/8th %) pilocarpine

1224. MC cause of Bilateral Horner's syndrome: Diabetes mellitus

1225. MC cause of congenital Horner's syndrome:
   I. Birth trauma
   II. Early cardiothoracic surgery

1226. MC mechanism of injury in congenital Horner's syndrome: Injury of the sympathetic plexus along its course in the neck or near the thoracic outlet

1227. MC central cause of a Horner syndrome: Lateral medullary stroke (Wallenberg syndrome)

1228. MC error that the ophthalmologist can make in the evaluation of the Horner syndrome:
   I. Imaging the head only and forgetting about the extracranial components of the oculosympathetic pathway
   II. To order a computed tomography (CT) scan alone as the MRI is more sensitive for the detection of the extracranial carotid dissection than the CT scan

MOST COMMONS IN OPHTHALMOLOGY

III. Not realizing the urgency of evaluation for an acute Horner syndrome as patients with an internal carotid dissection might suffer an ipsilateral hemispheric stroke from thromboembolic disease or have a potentially treatable dissection that requires emergent evaluation

1229. MC cause of painful postganglionic Horner syndrome: Traumatic or spontaneous dissection of the cervical internal carotid artery (ICA)

1230. MC finding in patients with ICA dissection: Acute isolated painful Horner's syndrome

1231. MC tumors causing preganglionic Horner's syndrome: Lung and Breast cancer

1232. MC site of injury for an iatrogenic Horner syndrome: Preganglionic neuron

1233. MC used pharmacologic agents for confirmation of Horner's syndrome: Cocaine and apraclonidine

1234. MC ocular manifestation of whiplash syndrome: Horner's syndrome

1235. MC cause of midposition (3-6 mm) fixed pupils: Mesencephalic damage from transtentorial herniation

1236. MC cause of Paradoxical Pupils (pupillary constriction in response to darkness):

    I.   Retinal dystrophies

    II.   Optic neuropathies

1237. MC causes of transient unilateral mydriasis:

    I.   Migraine

    II.   Benign episodic mydriasis

1238. MC complaint of patients with Benign episodic pupillary mydriasis or "springing pupil": Mild blur with photophobia

1239. MC people susceptible for Benign episodic pupillary mydriasis: Young women with migraines

Nystagmus & Related Disorders

1240. MC cause of Convergence retraction nystagmus: Pinealoma

1241. MC cause of pendular convergence nystagmus: CNS Whipple's disease

1242. MC cause of Dissociated (disjunctive) nystagmus: Internuclear ophthalmoplegia (INO)

1243. MC type of nystagmus:

    I.   Vertical nystagmus (Direction)

MOST COMMONS IN OPHTHALMOLOGY

　　II.　Manifest latent nystagmus

1244. MC type of infantile fixation instability: Infantile Nystagmus (IN)

1245. MC benign nystagmus seen in infancy:

　　I.　Infantile nystagmus syndrome (INS) also known as congenital nystagmus

　　II.　Fusion maldevelopment nystagmus syndrome (FMNS) also known as latent/manifest latent nystagmus

　　III.　Spasmus nutans syndrome (SNS)

　　IV.　Nystagmus blockage syndrome (NBS)

1246. MC waveform cycle in congenital nystagmus:

　　I.　Jerk

　　II.　Jerk with extended foveation

　　III.　Pendular

　　IV.　Pseudo-cycloid

1247. MC cause of dissociated jerk nystagmus: Internuclear ophthalmoplegia

1248. MC cause of Acquired Pendular Nystagmus (APN):

　　I.　Lesions due to multiple sclerosis

　　II.　Infarctions at different sites of the brainstem

MOST COMMONS IN OPHTHALMOLOGY

1249. MC cause of dissociated or ataxic nystagmus: Internuclear ophthalmoplegia (INO)

1250. MC ocular motor defect in patients with pontine infarcts: Internuclear ophthalmoplegia (INO)

1251. MC cause of upbeat nystagmus:

    I.   Cerebellar degeneration

    II.   Brainstem or Cerebellar Stroke

    III.   Demyelination and Tumors

1252. MC cause of torsional nystagmus:

    I.   Infarction

    II.   Multiple sclerosis

1253. MC type of nystagmus encountered in clinical practice: Gaze evoked nystagmus

1254. MC cause of gaze evoked nystagmus: Medications (Sedatives or anticonvulsants)

1255. MC feature of Spasmus nutans: Nystagmoid movements

1256. MC cause of unilateral horizontal nystagmus in infancy: Spasmus nutans

1257. MC cause of acquired see saw nystagmus: Parasellar mass

1258. MC type of strabismus in children with see saw nystagmus: Exotropia

1259. MC cause of downbeat nystagmus:

    I.   Developmental anomalies of the posterior fossa

    II.   Cerebellar degenerations

    III.   Multiple sclerosis

    IV.   Vertebrobasilar infarction

1260. MC neuro-ophthalmic sign occurring in patients with tumors of the spinal cord: Nystagmus

1261. MC diagnostic error in the evaluation of infantile nystagmus: Acquisition of neuroimaging studies in the child who is otherwise neurologically normal

1262. MC cause type of physiologic nystagmus: Unsustained end-point nystagmus

1263. MC cause of oscillopsia (Illusory movement of the environment): Rhythmic to-and-fro movements of the eyes (nystagmus)

1264. MC cause of monocular oscillopsia: Superior oblique myokymia

1265. MC feature of Spasmus nutans: Nystagmoid movements

1266. MC cause of unilateral horizontal nystagmus in infancy: Spasmus nutans

1267. MC condition associated with head nodding in children: Spasmus nutans

1268. MC form of positional nystagmus: Benign Paroxysmal Positional Vertigo (BPPV)

1269. MC semicircular canal affected in BPPV: Posterior semicircular canal

1270. MC specific etiology of BPPV: Head trauma

1271. MC cause of dizziness after head trauma: BPPV

1272. MC cause of Vertigo:

    I. Benign Paroxysmal Positional Vertigo

    II. Acute Peripheral Vestibulopathy

1273. MC reason for surgery in a case of infantile nystagmus syndrome (formerly known as congenital motor nystagmus): Compensatory head posture due to an eccentric null zone

1274. MC stimulus used to produce OKN: Pattern of black and white stripes presented on a rotating drum or moving tape

1275. MC non-nystagmic abnormal eye movement:

    I. Ocular flutter (involuntary horizontal saccades)

    II. Opsoclonus (involuntary saccades in all directions of gaze)

1276. MC cause of opsoclonus:

    I. Children: Neuroblastoma

    II. Young adults: Demyelinating disease

III. Elderly: Paraneoplastic syndromes

Optic Disc Related Disorders

1277. MC cause of increased intracranial pressure: Primary (or idiopathic) intracranial hypertension

1278. MC cause of pseudopapilledema:

   I. Hyperaemic, small, crowded disc of hyperopia

   II. Hyaloid remnants

   III. Optic disc drusen

   IV. Congenital disc elevations without visible drusen

   V. Myelinated nerve fibers

1279. MC cause of pseudopapilledema in children: Intrapapillary drusen

1280. MC nonvisual symptom of papilledema: Headache

1281. MC cause of papilledema: Primary intracranial hypertension or IIH (Idiopathic Intracranial Hypertension)

1282. MC cause of intracranial hypertension: IIH (Idiopathic Intracranial Hypertension)

1283. MC symptoms of IIH (Idiopathic Intracranial Hypertension):

MOST COMMONS IN OPHTHALMOLOGY

    I.   Headache: 90% (bifrontal or generalized, pressure-like, and often associated with neck pain)

    II.   Transient visual obscurations: 70%

    III.   Pulsatile tinnitus

    IV.   Diplopia: 40%

1284. MC examination finding in patients with raised ICP: Papilledema

1285. MC symptom of patients with raised ICP: Headache

1286. MC vascular problem causing Raised ICP: Cerebral sinovenous thrombosis

1287. MC visual field abnormalities in optic disc swelling:

    I.   Blind spot enlargement

    II.   Generalized constriction of isopters

    III.   Inferior nasal field loss

1288. MC type of meningitis causing papilledema:

    I.   Tuberculous meningitis

    II.   Cryptococcal meningitis

1289. MC tumors associated with childhood papilledema:

    I.   Midbrain and cerebellar glioma

    II.   Medulloblastoma

III. Ependymoma

1290. MC recognized causes of childhood IIH:

   I. Dural venous thrombosis

   II. Steroid withdrawal

   III. Malnutrition associated with refeeding

1291. MC cause of vision loss in optic disc pit: Serous detachment of macula

1292. MC location of optic disc pit: Inferotemporal disc

1293. MC visual field defect in optic disc pit: Para-central arcuate scotoma connected to an enlarged blind spot

1294. MC cause of optic neuritis:

   I. Demyelinating disorders like multiple sclerosis

   II. Viral (mumps, measles, herpes zoster, cytomegalovirus, or HIV)

   III. Bacterial (tuberculosis, syphilis or lymes disease)

   IV. Other (histoplasmosis, cryptococcosis, toxoplasmosis or toxocariasis)

1295. MC presentation of optic neuritis in adults: Retrobulbar neuritis (RBN)

1296. MC cause of Retrobulbar Neuritis (RBN): Multiple sclerosis

1297. MC CFS abnormalities in patients with Multiple Sclerosis:

I. Elevation of immunoglobulin G (igg) level
II. Elevation of the igg/albumin index
III. Presence of oligoclonal igg bands

1298. MC visual field defect in patients with optic neuritis: Diffuse suppression of the visual field on automated perimetry

1299. MC residual visual deficits in patients with resolved optic neuritis: Defective colour vision (tested with Farnsworth–Munsell 100-hue colour test)

1300. MC type of optic neuritis throughout the world: Acute Idiopathic Demyelinating Optic Neuritis

1301. MC type of tilt seen in tilted disc: Superotemporal downward tilt (so that the upper border of the disc appears elevated and the lower border appears flat and pale)

1302. MC visual field defect seen in the congenital tilted disc syndrome: Superior bitemporal defect not respecting the vertical meridian

1303. MC electrophysiological abnormality observed in the congenital tilted disc syndrome: Delayed latency or no response in the pattern reversal VEP

1304. MC syndrome of toxic damage to the optic nerve/chiasm: Tobacco–alcohol amblyopia

1305. MC cause of unilateral optic disc edema with a macular star (ODEMS): Cat scratch neuroretinitis

1306. MC congenital optic anomaly encountered in paediatric ophthalmic practice: Optic nerve hypoplasia (6.3 out of 100,000 children)

1307. MC endocrinologic abnormality associated with optic nerve hypoplasia/septo-optic dysplasia: Growth hormone deficiency

1308. MC segmental form of optic nerve hypoplasia encountered in clinical practice: Colobomas

1309. MC nonocular abnormalities associated with congenital optic nerve hypoplasia: Midline CNS structural defect

1310. MC associated finding with optic nerve aplasia: Colobomas

1311. MC cause of disc elevation: Optic disc drusen

1312. MC orbital cause of disc edema: Graves' orbitopathy

1313. MC cause of superior segment disc hypoplasia: Children of diabetic mothers

1314. MC cause of acquired pit in optic nerve head: Glaucoma

1315. MC visual field defects in optic neuritis on manual kinetic perimetry and tangent screen testing: Central scotoma

1316. MC visual field abnormality in optic neuritis on Humphrey 30-2 program: Decreased sensitivity over the entire central visual field

1317. MC differential diagnosis of diabetic papillopathy:

    I.   Optic disc neovascularization

    II.   Papilledema associated with elevated intracranial pressure

1318. MC infectious cause of optic neuritis: Viral

    I.   Direct viral infection (measles, rubella, mumps, chickenpox, influenza, CMV)

    II.   Postviral syndrome (postinfectious encephalomyelitis)

    III.   Postvaccination (mumps, measles, rubella)

1319. MC complication of Optic nerve sheath fenestration:

    I.   Diplopia from transient lateral rectus palsy

    II.   Pupillary dilation resulting from sphincter denervation

1320. MC complication associated with lumboperitoneal (LP) shunts:

    I.   Obstruction (account for up to 65% of all revisions)

    II.   Secondary intracranial hypotension caused by excessive drainage of CSF

1321. MC complication of the morning glory disc anomaly: Serous retinal detachment

1322. MC ocular findings of IRVAN (idiopathic retinal vasculitis, aneurysms, and neuroretinitis): Aneurysmal dilatations of the retinal and optic nerve head arterioles

1323. MC causes of congenital band atrophy of disc in children:
    I. Unilateral porencephaly
    II. Arteriovenous malformation
    III. Ganglioneuroma which involve the occipital lobe and lead to transsynaptic degeneration

1324. MC expression of segmental optic atrophy: Temporal pallor

1325. MC cause of unilateral optic disc swelling without visual loss: Orbital disease

1326. MC variety of crescent in disc: Inferior conus or Fuchs' coloboma

1327. MC cause of chronic unilateral disc swelling: Obstruction of the sub-arachnoid space of the ipsilateral nerve by an intraorbital process

Ischemic Optic Neuropathy

1328. MC acute optic neuropathies in patients older than 50 years: Ischemic optic neuropathies (IONs) (NAION in particular)

1329. MC type of IONs (Ischemic optic neuropathies): Nonarteritic Anterior Ischemic Optic Neuropathy (NAION)

1330. MC field defect in Nonarteritic Anterior Ischemic Optic Neuropathy (NAION):
    I. Inferior altitudinal (relative inferior altitudinal defect with absolute inferior nasal defect, inferior field being affected three times more commonly than the superior field)
    II. Superior altitudinal
    III. Arcuate

1331. MC topographic location of pallor of optic disc in NAION: Superior half of the disc

1332. MC time when NAION develops: Early morning during sleep

1333. MC cause of NAION:
    I. Transient nonperfusion or hypoperfusion of the optic nerve head circulation

II. Embolic lesions of the arteries/arterioles feeding the optic nerve head

1334. MC cause of carotid artery stenosis or occlusion and consequent development of NAION: Atherosclerotic changes in arteries

1335. MC cause of PION (Posterior Ischemic Optic Neuropathy):
   I. Giant cell arteritis
   II. Related to surgery (intraoperative hypotension during coronary artery bypass and lumbar spine procedures)

1336. MC visual field defect in PION (Posterior Ischemic Optic Neuropathy): Central visual field defect (central scotoma)

1337. MC underlying cause of AION: Hypertension

1338. MC etiology of vision loss in patient with GCA: Arteritic AION (Anterior Ischemic Optic Neuropathy)

1339. MC blood vessel involved in AAION caused by GCA: Medial PCA (posterior ciliary arteries) supplying retrolaminar and laminar regions

1340. MC associated disease with Arteritic Anterior Ischemic Optic Neuropathy (AAION): Giant cell arteritis (GCA)

MOST COMMONS IN OPHTHALMOLOGY

1341. MC ophthalmic manifestation of giant cell arteritis: Sudden unilateral visual loss due to anterior ischaemic optic neuropathy (AION) caused by occlusive inflammation in the posterior ciliary arteries

1342. MC symptom of Giant Cell Arteritis (GCA):
   I. Headache (Temporal > Occipital)
   II. Jaw claudication

1343. MC cause of death in patients with Giant Cell Arteritis: Cerebrovascular diseases

1344. MC ocular symptom of GCA:
   I. Vision loss (Partial or Complete)
   II. Diplopia

1345. MC etiology of vision loss in patient with GCA:
   I. Arteritic AION (Anterior Ischemic Optic Neuropathy)
   II. Central retinal artery occlusion

1346. MC neurologic complication of GCA: Peripheral neuropathy

1347. MC cranial nerve involved in GCA: Oculomotor nerve (usually sparing the pupil)

1348. MC pupillary abnormality associated with GCA:
   I. Relative APD (RAPD)

MOST COMMONS IN OPHTHALMOLOGY

    II.   Tonic pupil

    III.   Horner's syndrome

1349. MC involved blood vessels in GCA:

    I.   Superficial temporal artery

    II.   Occipital artery

    III.   Vertebral artery

    IV.   Ophthalmic artery

    V.   Posterior ciliary artery

1350. MC blood vessel involved in AAION caused by GCA: Medial PCA (posterior ciliary arteries) supplying retrolaminar and laminar regions

1351. MC cause of amaurosis fugax in GCA: Transient ischemia of the ONH

1352. MC histopathologic testing for GCA: Temporal artery biopsy

1353. MC mechanism of arteritic ION: Sudden optic nerve infarction due to vessel lumens narrowed by vasculitis

1354. MC cause of optic atrophy on one side and optic disc swelling on the other side: Bilateral nonsimultaneous optic neuritis

1355. MC cause of Hypotensive Ischemic Optic Neuropathy: Cardiac bypass or prolonged lumbar spine surgery

Other Optic Neuropathies

1356. MC optic neuropathy: Glaucoma

1357. MC acute optic neuropathy in young and middle-aged adults: Optic Neuritis

1358. MC hereditary optic neuropathy:

    I.   Dominant optic atrophy (DOA) or Kjer's disease (1 in 50000)

    II.   Leber's hereditary optic neuropathy (LHON)

1359. MC cause of optic neuropathy of malnutrition: Deficiency of vitamin B12

1360. MC cause of light-near dissociation (LND): Optic neuropathy

1361. MC cardiac abnormalities found in patients with Leber's hereditary optic neuropathy (LHON):

    I.   Wolff Parkinson White Syndrome

    II.   Lown Ganong Levine Syndrome

1362. MC causes of optic neuropathy in young adults: Inflammatory optic neuropathies

1363. MC fungal cause of optic neuropathy: Cryptococcus

1364. MC primary carcinoma sites causing carcinomatous optic neuropathy: Lung and breast

MOST COMMONS IN OPHTHALMOLOGY

1365. MC type of paraneoplastic process causing vision loss: Paraneoplastic optic neuropathy (PON)

1366. MC identified paraneoplastic antibody: CV2/CRMP-5

1367. MC tumor causing Paraneoplastic optic neuropathy (PON):
    I. Small cell carcinoma of the lung
    II. Thymoma

1368. MC cause of late visual deterioration after CNS tumor excision and radiation: Tumor recurrence

1369. MC recognized nutritional or toxic optic neuropathy: Tobacco–alcohol amblyopia

1370. MC visual field defects seen in nutritional or toxic optic neuropathies:
    I. Central scotomas
    II. Cecocentral scotomas

1371. MC cause of Radiation optic neuropathy (RON): Irradiation of pituitary adenoma

1372. MC cranial neuropathy in Sphenoid Wing Meningioma: Optic neuropathy

1373. MC inflammatory etiology of infiltrative optic neuropathies: Sarcoidosis

1374. MC reported causes of blood loss associated with Ischemic Optic Neuropathy (ION):

MOST COMMONS IN OPHTHALMOLOGY

    I. Spontaneous gastrointestinal or uterine bleeding

    II. Surgically induced haemorrhage, related most frequently to cardiac bypass or lumbar spine procedures

1375. MC identified lesions causing retrobulbar compressive optic neuropathy without disc swelling:

    I. Meningiomas

    II. Pituitary Tumors

    III. Aneurysms

1376. MC lesions causing Infiltrative Optic Neuropathy:

    I. Primary Tumors: Optic glioma

    II. Secondary Tumors: Metastatic carcinoma

    III. Inflammatory disorders: Sarcoidosis

    IV. Infectious agents: Opportunistic fungi

1377. MC drug causing Toxic optic neuropathy: Ethambutol

1378. MC symptom of ethambutol related optic neuropathy: Blue-yellow colour changes

1379. MC toxin causing Toxic Optic Neuropathy: Methanol

1380. MC cause of blindness secondary to thyroid orbitopathy: Optic neuropathy

1381. MC cause of Syndrome of Chronic Optic Nerve Compression:

Sphenorbital meningiomas

Brainstem Disorders

1382. MC ischemic lesion of the brainstem: Lateral medulla infarction

(Wallenberg's syndrome)

1383. MC cause of Wallenberg's Lateral Medullary Syndrome: Thrombotic

occlusion of the ipsilateral vertebral artery

1384. MC type of nystagmus in Wallenberg's Lateral Medullary Syndrome:

Torsional nystagmus

1385. MC clinical signs of Wallenberg's Lateral Medullary Syndrome:

   I.   Ataxia

   II. Numbness of the face and/or body

   III. Horner's syndrome

1386. MC cause of one-and-a-half syndrome:

   I.   Brainstem infarction

   II. Multiple sclerosis

   III. Pontine haemorrhage

   IV. Tumors

1387. MC cause of Eight-and-a-half syndrome (7+1.5=8.5, lesion producing the one-and-a-half syndrome but also involving the intra-axial portion of the facial nerve): Stroke

1388. MC sign of intrinsic brainstem damage: Ocular tilt reaction

1389. MC causes of brainstem damage:
    I.   Demyelinating diseases (multiple sclerosis) in the young
    II. Ischemic vascular disease in the elderly

1390. MC cause of ocular tilt reaction in adults: Acute vascular brainstem stroke

1391. MC cause of ocular tilt reaction in children: Posterior fossa tumors

1392. MC encountered brainstem tumor in children: Diffuse gliomas

1393. MC site of origin of brainstem gliomas:
    I.   Pons
    II. Midbrain
    III. Medulla

1394. MC etiology of dorsal midbrain syndrome:
    I.   Pineal gland cyst or haemorrhage or pinealoma
    II. Hydrocephalus

MOST COMMONS IN OPHTHALMOLOGY

1395. MC eye movement abnormality in dorsal midbrain syndrome: Upgaze saccadic palsy

1396. MC eyelid abnormality in dorsal midbrain syndrome: Eyelid retraction (Collier's tucked lid sign)

1397. MC cause of convergence paralysis: Dorsal midbrain syndrome

1398. MC cause of Convergence retraction nystagmus: Pinealoma

1399. MC cause of pendular convergence nystagmus: CNS Whipple's disease

1400. MC lesion producing the "Parinaud-plus" syndrome: Pinealomas

1401. MC sign of pinealoma: Papilledema

1402. MC symptom of pinealoma: Headache

1403. MC brain stem disturbance that causes a horizontal gaze deficit: Lesion in the pons

1404. MC cause of pontine horizontal gaze palsy:

    I. Older patients: Ischemia due to atherosclerosis

    II. Younger patients: Demyelinating processes (multiple sclerosis)

    III. Children: Pontine gliomas or medulloblastomas

1405. MC cause of supranuclear downgaze paresis: Vascular insult involving a paramedian artery of the mesencephalon and thalamus

Internuclear Ophthalmoplegia

1406. MC horizontal eye movement paralysis: Internuclear ophthalmoparesis (INO)

1407. MC presentation of internuclear ophthalmoplegia (INO): Impaired adduction of one eye associated with monocular nystagmus in the contralateral (abducting) eye

1408. MC ocular motor disturbance of demyelinative origin: Internuclear ophthalmoplegia (INO)

1409. MC cause of central lateral gaze paralysis: Internuclear ophthalmoparesis (INO)

1410. MC cause of cause of unilateral internuclear ophthalmoplegia: Infarct of a small branch of the basilar artery

1411. MC cause of Internuclear ophthalmoparesis (INO):
    I. Multiple sclerosis (in younger patients)
    II. Vascular lesions such as infarction, haemorrhage, and arteriovenous malformations (in older patients)
    III. Tumors

1412. MC mechanism of INO: Disruption of the ipsilateral medial longitudinal fasciculus (MLF)

1413. MC mechanism of MLF lesion in an elderly: Infarct

1414. MC type of vestibular cell projecting to the vertical oculomotor motor nuclei through the MLF: Tonic-vestibular-pause (TVP) cells (aka position-vestibular-pause or PVP cells)

1415. MC cause of cause of bilateral internuclear ophthalmoplegia: Multiple sclerosis

1416. MC cause of dissociated jerk nystagmus: Internuclear ophthalmoplegia

1417. MC cause of dissociated or ataxic nystagmus: Internuclear ophthalmoplegia (INO)

1418. MC ocular motor defect in patients with pontine infarcts: Internuclear ophthalmoplegia (INO)

Neuromuscular Disorders

1419. MC presenting signs of myasthenia gravis: Ocular sign

1420. MC presentation of ocular myasthenia:

    I.   Ptosis

    II. Diplopia

1421. MC elicited sign for myasthenia evaluation: Lid fatigue on prolonged up gaze

1422. MC cause of Cogan's lid twitch sign (upper eyelid retracts momentarily due to an overshoot following an upward saccade from downgaze): Myasthenia gravis

1423. MC muscles affected in Ocular myasthenia:
    I.   Levator
    II. Extraocular muscles
    III. Orbicularis oculi

1424. MC autoimmune disorder associated with ocular myasthenia: Thyroid eye disease

1425. MC confirmatory test utilised for myasthenia: The Tensilon (edrophonium hydrochloride) test

1426. MC used steroid sparing immunosuppressant for myasthenia gravis: Azathioprine

1427. MC myogenic palsy seen in ophthalmic departments: Myasthenia gravis

1428. MC disease of the neuromuscular junction (NMJ): Myasthenia gravis (MG)

1429. MC used immunomodulatory treatment for myasthenia gravis:

Corticosteroids

1430. MC associated abnormality with Myasthenia Gravis: Thymic tumors or thymic hyperplasia

1431. MC associated cancer with Lambert-Eaton myasthenic syndrome: Small cell lung cancer

1432. MC mutations in congenital myasthenic syndromes:
   I. Mutations that reduce the expression or alter the kinetics of the acetylcholine receptor
   II. Mutations of the acetylcholinesterase molecule

1433. MC cause of ocular neuromyotonia: Prior radiation to the orbit or sellar region for parasellar, sinus or skull base tumors

Intracranial Vascular Disorders

1434. MC type of intracranial aneurysm: Saccular or "berry" aneurysm

1435. MC manifestation of intracranial aneurysms: Subarachnoid Haemorrhage

MOST COMMONS IN OPHTHALMOLOGY

1436. MC cause of subarachnoid haemorrhage in adults: Intracranial aneurysm

1437. MC cause of subarachnoid haemorrhage in children: Arteriovenous malformation (AVM)

1438. MC mode of presentation of Arteriovenous Malformation:
    I. Subarachnoid haemorrhage
    II. Seizures

1439. MC cause of spontaneous intracranial haemorrhage in children: AV Malformations (AVM)

1440. MC abnormality of the intracranial circulation in childhood: AV Malformations (AVM)

1441. MC mode of performing stereotactic radiosurgery for intracranial AVMs: Gamma knife

1442. MC cause of intense and incapacitating headache of abrupt onset: Subarachnoid haemorrhage (SAH)

1443. MC single location of intracranial aneurysm: Anterior Communicating Artery

1444. MC presentation of cerebral venous sinus thrombosis (CVT): New onset of headache with a focal neurologic deficit or a partial seizure

MOST COMMONS IN OPHTHALMOLOGY

1445. MC cause of Homonymous hemianopia:

   I.   Adults: Stroke (infarction of the calcarine cortex with occlusion of the posterior cerebral artery or its branches)

   II. Children: Trauma and Tumors

1446. MC cause of ischemic stroke: Embolism

1447. MC cause of persistent cerebral blindness: Cerebrovascular infarction

1448. MC cause of pure alexia: Left posterior cerebral artery ischemia

1449. MC nerve involved in ophthalmoplegic migraine: Third nerve

1450. MC neuro-ophthalmic presentation associated with an aneurysm at the junction of the internal carotid and posterior communicating artery: Pupil-involving 3rd nerve palsy

1451. MC cause of an occipital lobe hemianopia in adults: PCA stroke

1452. MC presentation of a PCA stroke: Homonymous hemianopia, with or without macular sparing

1453. MC neuro-ophthalmologic manifestation of an unruptured MCA aneurysm: Contralateral homonymous visual field defect

1454. MC organism implicated in Septic thrombosis of the cavernous sinuses: Staphylococcus aureus

MOST COMMONS IN OPHTHALMOLOGY

1455. MC tumors to cause cavernous sinus syndrome: Nasopharyngeal carcinomas

1456. MC cause of cavernous sinus lesions: Cavernous sinus meningiomas

1457. MC nerve affected in cavernous sinus syndrome:

    I.   6th CN

    II.   5th CN

    III.   3rd CN

    IV.   4th CN

    V.   Optic nerve

1458. MC pathogens that produce odontogenic septic thrombosis of the cavernous sinus:

    I.   Streptococci

    II.   Fusobacteria

    III.   Bacteroides

1459. MC nerve affected in Tolosa–Hunt syndrome:

    I.   3rd CN

    II.   4th CN

    III.   5th CN

    IV.   6th CN

MOST COMMONS IN OPHTHALMOLOGY

1460. MC classification used to describe CCF: Barrow classification

1461. MC cause of direct Carotid–Cavernous Fistula (CCF): Severe trauma

1462. MC cause of indirect Carotid–Cavernous Fistula (CCF): Spontaneous rupture

1463. MC type of DAVFs (Dural Arteriovenous Fistulas): Fistulas draining into a sinus or a meningeal vein

1464. MC corneal sign encountered in patients with a direct CCF: Exposure keratopathy

1465. MC ocular motor nerve paresis that occurs in patients with a direct carotid-cavernous fistula: Abducens nerve paresis

1466. MC cause of glaucoma in patients with direct CCF: Increased episcleral venous pressure

1467. MC complaints of patients with carotid–cavernous fistulas (CCF):
    I. Subjective bruit (80%)
    II. Visual blur (59%)
    III. Headache (53%)
    IV. Diplopia (53%)
    V. Ocular or orbital pain (35%)

1468. MC coils used for closure of a direct CCF: Platinum detachable coils

1469. MC ocular signs of septic lateral sinus thrombosis: Abducens nerve paresis

1470. MC presentation of internal carotid artery dissection: Headache with ipsilateral ophthalmic signs and contralateral neurologic deficits

1471. MC locations involved by Cerebral Venous Thrombosis:

    I. Cavernous sinus

    II. Lateral (transverse) sinus

    III. Superior sagittal sinus

1472. MC ophthalmic signs of Lateral (transverse) sinus thrombosis: Papilledema and sixth nerve palsy

1473. MC laboratory finding in patient with cerebral venous thrombosis:

    I. Protein C deficiency

    II. Protein S deficiency

    III. Presence of antiphospholipid and anticardiolipin antibodies

    IV. Factor V Leiden

    V. Presence of prothrombin G20210A mutation

    VI. Hyperhomocysteinemia

1474. MC used neurointerventional technique for the treatment of aneurysms: Filling the aneurysm sac with embolic material, which is most often a controlled-release detachable platinum microcoil

1475. MC visual field defect associated with BAVM (Brain Arterio Vencus Malformations): Homonymous Hemianopia

1476. MC vascular malformation found within the pons: Telangiectasias

1477. MC affected area by Brain ArterioVenous Malformation (BAVMs):
   I.   Parietal lobe (27%)
   II. Frontal lobe (22%)

1478. MC visual field defect associated with BAVMs: Homonymous hemianopia

1479. MC vascular malformation found in pons: Telangiectasias

1480. MC intracranial vascular anomaly found at autopsy: Venous angiomas

Facial Nerve & Related Disorders

1481. MC cranial nerves damaged by perinatal injury: Facial nerve

1482. MC situations in which lacrimal pump failure is present despite patency of the membranous lacrimal conduit: Facial nerve paresis

1483. MC cranial nerve affected in SLE: Facial nerve

1484. MC cranial nerve involved in sarcoidosis:

    I.   Facial nerve

    II.   Optic nerve

1485. MC Disorders of Overactivity of the Seventh Nerve:

    I.   Essential blepharospasm

    II.   Hemifacial spasm (HFS)

    III.   Facial myokymia

1486. MC cause of Hemifacial spasm (HFS): Irritation of the seventh nerve roots by a dilated or tortuous vascular structure

1487. MC cause of Essential Blepharospasm: Disturbance of basal ganglia

1488. MC exacerbating factor for Benign essential blepharospasm (BEB): Light (so patients may find some relief with filtered glasses)

1489. MC offending vessel causing seventh nerve root irritation leading to hemifacial spasm (HFS):

    I.   anterior inferior cerebellar artery

    II.   posterior inferior cerebellar artery

    III.   Vertebral artery

1490. MC position of head that can help diminish or halt the hemifacial spasms (HFS): Contralateral lateral decubitus position

1491. MC associated tumor with hemifacial spasm: Congenital or acquired cholesteatoma

1492. MC neurologic association with hemifacial spasm: Trigeminal neuralgia

1493. MC diagnostic modality employed for hemifacial spasm: MRI with MRA of the Head and Neck

1494. MC persistent complications of posterior fossa microvascular decompression surgery for HFS:
    I.   Ipsilateral hearing loss (1–13%)
    II. Facial paralysis (1–6%)

1495. MC used medical therapy for HFS:
    I.   Carbamazepine (Tegretol)
    II. Diphenylhydantoin (Dilantin)
    III. Dimethylaminoethanol (Deanol)

1496. MC cause of recurrent alternating facial palsy: Melkersson-Rosenthal syndrome

1497. MC cause of bilateral simultaneous facial palsy: Guillain-Barré syndrome

1498. MC ophthalmic treatment for facial palsy: Use of frequent lubricants

1499. MC cause of acute facial palsy: Bell's palsy

1500. MC mechanism of Aberrant Facial Nerve Regeneration:

   I.   Wallerian degeneration of axons with resultant abnormal branching during axonal regeneration

   II. Nuclear hyperexcitability

   III. Central cortex reorganization

1501. MC cause of Facial myokymia: Multiple sclerosis and brainstem glioma

1502. MC type of facial myokymia: Eyelid myokymia involving lower eyelid

Intracranial Tumors

1503. MC primary malignancies causing intracranial metastasis:

   I. Lung carcinoma (40% metastasize to the brain)

   II. Breast carcinoma (roughly 25 percent metastasize to the brain)

1504. MC type of craniopharyngiomas: Adamantinomatous

1505. MC space-occupying diseases of the sellar region:

   I. Pituitary adenoma

   II. Craniopharyngiomas

1506. MC sellar masses in children:

   I. Chiasmal/hypothalamic gliomas

MOST COMMONS IN OPHTHALMOLOGY

II. Craniopharyngiomas

1507. MC brain tumors of nonglial origin in children: Craniopharyngiomas

1508. MC supratentorial tumour in children: Craniopharyngiomas

1509. MC presentation of craniopharyngioma: Superiorly growth into ventricles leading to hydrocephalus and raised intracranial pressure

1510. MC surgical treatment of hydrocephalus:
   I. Ventriculoperitoneal shunts
   II. Endoscopic third ventriculostomy

1511. MC intracranial tumor: Pituitary adenoma

1512. MC intracranial tumor to extend into the orbit: Meningioma

1513. MC ophthalmological sign of a pituitary adenoma: Bitemporal loss of visual field

1514. MC pituitary tumors:
   I. Prolactinomas (35%)
   II. Somatotropin-secreting tumors (25%)
   III. Adrenocorticotrophic hormone (ACTH)-producing tumors (5%)

1515. MC cause of hypopituitarism in adults: Prolactinoma

1516. MC cause of hypopituitarism in children: Craniopharyngioma

MOST COMMONS IN OPHTHALMOLOGY

1517. MC ophthalmic sign of brain metastases: Papilledema caused by obstruction of CSF flow

1518. MC form of meningioma:
    I. Meningothelial
    II. Fibrous
    III. Transitional

1519. MC misdiagnosis of tuberculum sellae meningiomas: Recurrent optic neuritis

1520. MC initial symptom of Sphenoid Wing Meningioma: Slowly progressive unilateral proptosis

1521. MC cranial neuropathy in Sphenoid Wing Meningioma: Optic neuropathy

1522. MC visual field defects in Sphenoid Wing Meningioma:
    I. Temporal hemianopias
    II. Superior temporal defects
    III. Inferior temporal defects

1523. MC disease affecting orbital bones: Sphenoid wing meningioma

1524. MC tumor spreading from intracranial space to orbit: Sphenoid Meningioma

1525. MC metastatic tumors to the optic nerve: Breast and lung tumors

MOST COMMONS IN OPHTHALMOLOGY

1526. MC affected calvarial bone in fibrous dysplasia (FD):

  I.   frontal bone

  II. sphenoid

  III. temporal

  IV. parietal

  V.   occipital bones

1527. MC presentation of fibrous dysplasia (FD): Painless enlargement of the involved bone, causing facial asymmetry, orbital dystopia, or unilateral proptosis

1528. MC orbital wall involved by Fibrous Dysplasia: Roof of the orbit

1529. MC subtype of fibrous dysplasia (FD): Monostotic form (70-80%)

1530. MC histopathological pattern of Fibrous dysplasia of craniofacial bones:

  I.   Pagetoid pattern (56%)

  II. Sclerotic (23%)

  III. Cystlike (21%)

1531. MC bone involved by Juvenile ossifying fibroma of the orbit:

  I.   Orbital roof

  II. Ethmoid bone

  III. Maxilla

MOST COMMONS IN OPHTHALMOLOGY

1532. MC visual symptom in patients with olfactory groove meningiomas: Loss of central vision

1533. MC visual signs in patients with olfactory groove meningiomas:
    I.   Papilledema
    II. Optic atrophy

1534. MC primary tumor that involves the corpus callosum: Lipoma

1535. MC site of intracranial lipoma: Corpus callosum

1536. MC site of choroid plexus papillomas in children: Lateral ventricles

1537. MC site of choroid plexus papillomas in adults: 4th ventricle

1538. MC site of intracranial teratoma: Pineal region

1539. MC ocular motor nerve affected by Schwannoma:
    I.   Oculomotor nerve
    II. Trochlear nerve
    III. Abducens nerve

1540. MC cranial nerve affected by multiple myeloma: Abducens nerve

1541. MC lesion of the CNS occurring in patients with Von Hippel-Lindau Disease (VHLD): Hemangioblastomas

1542. MC location for hemangioblastomas associated with von Hippel–Lindau (VHL) disease: Cerebellum

1543. MC cause of death in von Hippel–Lindau (VHL) disease:

    I.   Cerebellar hemangioblastoma

    II.   Renal cell carcinoma

1544. MC ocular manifestation of von Hippel–Lindau (VHL) disease: Retinal capillary hemangiomas (RCH)

1545. MC location of retinal capillary hemangioma in VHL disease:

    I.   temporal equatorial region

    II.   on the optic nerve

1546. MC observed ocular sign of frontal lobe tumors: Papilledema

Misc Neuro-ophthalmology

1547. MC ocular manifestation of multiple sclerosis:

    I.   optic neuritis

    II.   internuclear ophthalmoplegia

    III.   nystagmus

1548. MC cause of Terson's syndrome:

    I.   ruptured anterior communicating aneurysms

    II.   Subarachnoid haemorrhage

1549. MC source of origin of retention mucocele:

I. frontal paranasal sinuses
   II. ethmoidal paranasal sinuses

1550. MC hormone receptors expressed by meningioma cells: Estrogen and progesterone receptors

1551. MC site of Schwannomas:
   I. vestibular division of the eighth cranial nerve
   II. trigeminal nerve root

1552. MC site of origin of orbital schwanommas: Superior ciliary nerves

1553. MC etiology of cerebral achromatopsia: Embolic stroke in the territory of the PCA

1554. MC cause of palinopsia: Parieto-occipital damage involving either hemisphere (MC Right hemisphere)

1555. MC form of dysmetropsia (visual illusion): Micropsia

1556. MC group of patients experiencing Erythropsia (pronounced shift of colour perception toward the long-wavelength end of the spectrum): Pseudophakic patients (whose eyes no longer have the yellow filter provided by the native lens of the ageing eye)

1557. MC acquired dyschromatopsia associated with glaucoma: Acquired deficit of blue/yellow discrimination

MOST COMMONS IN OPHTHALMOLOGY

1558. MC ophthalmologic symptom of disease of the internal carotid arterial system: Transient monocular visual loss (TMVL)

1559. MC identifiable cause of transient monocular visual loss: Atheromatous disease affecting the internal carotid or ophthalmic arteries

1560. MC cause of transient binocular visual disturbance: Migraine

1561. MC neuro-ophthalmic manifestation of Chiari syndrome: Downbeat nystagmus

1562. MC type of Chiari malformation presenting in childhood: Chiari Type I (Chiari type II was most common until recently)

1563. MC cause of unilateral orbicularis weakness: VII nerve (Bell's) palsy

1564. MC ocular motor pattern in Möbius syndrome:
    I. bilateral 6th nerve palsy
    II. bilateral horizontal gaze palsies

1565. MC anomaly in Gaucher's disease: Oculomotor apraxia

1566. MC presentation of thalamic stroke:
    I. impaired upgaze
    II. combination of impaired upgaze and downgaze

1567. MC pathology in Cogan's Congenital Ocular Motor Apraxia (COMA):
    I. agenesis of the corpus callosum

II. cerebellar hypoplasia

III. dilation of the fourth ventricle

1568. MC source of a locally derived brain abscess: Untreated or incompletely treated middle ear infection

1569. MC examples of abnormal cranial nerve synkineses:

I. Duane's Retraction Syndrome (DRS)

II. Marcus Gunn jaw-winking phenomenon (trigemino-ocular motor synkinesis)

1570. MC type of congenital neurogenic synkinetic ptosis: Marcus Gunn (Jaw-Winking) ptosis (MGJWP)

1571. MC type of Marcus Gunn jaw-winking (trigemino-oculomotor synkinesis):

I. external pterygoid-levator synkinesis: Lid elevation when the jaw is projected forward, thrust to the opposite side, or opened widely

II. internal pterygoid-levator synkinesis: Lid elevation triggered by clenching of the teeth

1572. MC movement that causes elevation of the ptotic eyelid in MGJWP: Lateral mandibular movement to the contralateral side

MOST COMMONS IN OPHTHALMOLOGY

1573. MC ocular motor disturbances seen with patients of Marcus Gunn phenomenon:
    I. double elevator palsy
    II. unilateral superior rectus palsy
    III. Duane retraction syndrome
    IV. adduction palsy with synergistic divergence

1574. MC recognized form of oculomotor synkinesis: Lid retraction on adduction

1575. MC mechanism of oculomotor synkinesis:
    I. peripheral misdirection at the site of injury
    II. ephaptic transmission
    III. central reorganization of motoneurons and their inputs

1576. MC cause of bilateral visual impairment in children in the developed world: Cortical Visual Impairment (CVI)

1577. MC cause of CVI: Perinatal hypoxic-ischemic event

1578. MC EEG finding of CVI: Absence of the alpha rhythm, which normally develops by 3 months of age and is elicited by eye closure and extinguished by eye opening. (Patients with alpha rhythm tend to have more residual vision)

1579. MC cause of excessive CSF secretion: Papilloma of the choroid plexus

MOST COMMONS IN OPHTHALMOLOGY

1580. MC brain abnormality seen in premature infants following prolonged asphyxia: Periventricular necrosis

1581. MC cranial nerves damaged by perinatal injury: Facial nerve

1582. MC involved cranial nerves in paediatric meningitis: III, IV, and VI (presumably from inflammation of the perineurium)

1583. MC ophthalmologic sequelae of paediatric meningitis: Optic atrophy and cranial nerve palsy

1584. MC sequela of paediatric meningitis: Hearing loss

1585. MC neurodegenerative condition in children: Neuronal ceroid lipofuscinosis (NCL) (aka Batten's disease)

1586. MC type of Neuronal ceroid lipofuscinosis (NCL): Juvenile type (CLN 3, Spielmeyer–Vogt/ Batten disease)

1587. MC used procedure for prenatal diagnosis of Adrenoleukodystrophy: Measurement of VLCFA levels in chorionic villus or amniocyte samples

1588. MC paediatric disorder of mitochondrial function: Leigh syndrome

1589. MC organisms associated with congenital neurologic infection:
    I.   rubella
    II. cytomegalovirus (CMV)
    III. varicella

IV. toxoplasma

V. herpes simplex

1590. MC nonocular structure involved in myoclonus: Soft palate

1591. MC cause of chiasmal syndrome:

    I. pituitary adenoma

    II. parasellar meningioma

    III. craniopharyngioma

    IV. parasellar internal carotid artery aneurysm

1592. MC causes of retrochiasmal vision loss: Strokes and neoplasms

1593. MC relationship of the optic chiasm relative to the pituitary fossa:

    I. Directly above the pituitary fossa (~ 80%)

    II. Prefixed (~ 10%)

    III. Postfixed (~ 10%)

1594. MC neuro-ophthalmic presentation of a unilateral retrochiasmal disturbance: Homonymous hemianopic field defect with normal acuity

1595. MC cause of unilateral retrochiasmal visual loss in adults: Stroke

1596. MC cause of unilateral retrochiasmal visual loss in children:

    I. Tumors

    II. Trauma

MOST COMMONS IN OPHTHALMOLOGY

1597. MC causes of optic radiation hemianopias in adults:

   I. Strokes in the MCA distribution

   II. neoplasms

1598. MC cause of central visual impairment in preterm infants: Periventricular leukomalacia

1599. MC cause of central visual impairment in term infants: Hypoxic ischemic encephalopathy

1600. MC cause of alexia without agraphia: Posterior cerebral artery distribution stroke

1601. MC cause of prosopagnosia:

   I. posterior cerebral artery stroke (causing bilateral lesions involving the inferior temporo-occipital junction)

   II. head trauma

   III. viral encephalitis

1602. MC cause of the ischemic form of transient visual loss: Extracranial internal carotid artery stenosis or occlusion

1603. MC nonischemic causes of transient visual loss: Tear film or corneal abnormalities

1604. MC cause of palinopsia (trailing effect behind moving objects): Parieto-occipital damage with incomplete homonymous hemianopic field loss

1605. MC associated feature of Möbius syndrome (Congenital facial diplegia): Abducens palsy

1606. MC cause of Chiasmal radionecrosis: Irradiation of pituitary adenoma

1607. MC ocular complaint of Parkinson's disease (PD) patients: Decreased blink rate leading to ocular surface irritation (blepharitis)

1608. MC cause of oculopalatal tremor (OPT): Delayed consequence of strokes in the brainstem tegmentum or cerebellum

1609. MC ophthalmologic abnormality in Smith–Lemli–Opitz syndrome (SLOS): Blepharoptosis

1610. MC symptom of occipital lobe epilepsy: Elementary visual hallucinations

1611. MC early sign of progressive supranuclear palsy: Downgaze paresis

1612. MC causes of upgaze palsy in children:
    I. hydrocephalus (congenital and acquired)
    II. various conditions associated with the dorsal midbrain syndrome

1613. MC protein toxins responsible for human botulism: Protein A, B and E of Clostridium botulinum

MOST COMMONS IN OPHTHALMOLOGY

1614. MC ocular presenting symptom of botulism: Diplopia

1615. MC type of botulism: Infant botulism

1616. MC source of infection in Infant botulism: Contaminated honey

1617. MC neuroradiologic abnormality in Periodic alternating gaze deviation (PAGD): Cerebellar vermis atrophy

1618. MC location for arachnoid cysts: Middle cranial fossa

1619. MC cerebellar malformation associated with the PHACE (Posterior fossa malformations, Hemangiomas, Arterial malformations, Coarcation of the Aorta and other cardiac defects, and Eye abnormalities) syndrome: Dandy Walker syndrome

1620. MC neuro-ophthalmologic association of Gray Matter Heterotopia: Isolated optic nerve hypoplasia

1621. MC cranial nerve dysfunction associated with Acute haemorrhagic conjunctivitis caused by enterovirus 70:
    I. Solitary 7th nerve palsy
    II. Solitary 5th nerve palsy
    III. Combined 7th and 5th nerve palsy

1622. MC cause of diplopia from increased ICP: Lateral rectus palsy

MOST COMMONS IN OPHTHALMOLOGY

1623. MC etiologic factor producing cortical blindness: Hypoxia or ischemia of the occipital lobes

1624. MC cause of crocodile tears (Bogorad syndrome): On the side of a facial palsy with anomalous lacrimal gland innervation

1625. MC type of gustolacrimal reflex: Acquired Gustolacrimal Reflex Following Facial Palsy or Sectioning of the Greater Superficial Petrosal Nerve

1626. MC cause of Miller Fisher syndrome (triad of ophthalmoplegia, ataxia, and areflexia): Campylobacter jejuni infection (serotype 0-2 or 0-10)

1627. MC pupillary abnormality in Miller Fisher Syndrome: Unilateral or bilateral pupillary dilation with a poor or no reaction to light stimulation

1628. MC mechanism of Partial or complete oculomotor nerve dysfunction also may occur following dental anaesthesia: The anesthetic solution is inadvertently injected into the inferior dental artery or superior alveolar artery → retrograde flow into the maxillary artery → middle meningeal artery, the orbital branch of which forms a fairly constant anastomosis with the lacrimal branch of the ophthalmic artery

1629. MC mitochondrial syndromes in which ophthalmoplegia is a prominent feature:

MOST COMMONS IN OPHTHALMOLOGY

    I. Chronic progressive external ophthalmoplegia (CPEO)

    II. Kearns-Sayre syndrome (KSS)

1630. MC presenting syndrome of Kearns–Sayre syndrome: Ptosis (vision loss and a pigmentary retinopathy develops later)

1631. MC manifestation of mitochondrial myopathies: CPEO

1632. MC muscle involved in chronic progressive external ophthalmoplegia (CPEO): Medial rectus

1633. MC cause of apraxia of eyelid opening (AEO) (inability to initiate eyelid opening in the absence of visible orbicularis contraction and in the absence of paralysis):

    I. Progressive supranuclear palsy

    II. Parkinson disease

    III. Atypical parkinsonism

1634. MC eyelid disturbance in patients with Corticobasal Degeneration (CBD): Apraxia of lid opening

1635. MC causes of acquired neurogenic ptosis: Dysfunction of the oculomotor nucleus, fascicle, or nerve

1636. MC causes of myopathic insufficiency of eyelid closure:

    I. Congenital muscular dystrophy

II. Myotonic dystrophy

III. Mitochondrial cytopathies associated with CPEO

1637. MC causes of ocular blepharospasm:

   I. Disturbances of the eyelids (e.g., blepharitis, trichiasis, entropion)

   II. Disturbances of the corneal epithelium

   III. Severe dry eyes

   IV. Iritis, scleritis, and angle-closure glaucoma

1638. MC sensory deficit from orbital disease: Hypoesthesia in the territory of the supraorbital or supratrochlear nerve

1639. MC clinical symptom of intracranial hypotension: Headache

1640. MC cause of symptomatic intracranial hypotension: Lumbar puncture (LP)

1641. MC Neuro-ophthalmic manifestations of intracranial hypotension: Unilateral or bilateral sixth nerve palsies

1642. MC used treatment for persistent low-pressure headache: Epidural blood patch

1643. MC neuro-ophthalmologic manifestation of maple syrup urine disease: Ophthalmoplegia

1644. MC ocular manifestation of generalized and cephalic tetanus: Blepharospasm

1645. MC neuro-ophthalmologic manifestation of diphtheria: Paresis of accommodation

1646. MC parasitic disease of the central nervous system: Neurocysticercosis

1647. MC diagnosed form of cysticercosis: Neurocysticercosis

1648. MC cause of neurologic disease in patients with AIDS: CNS toxoplasmosis

1649. MC neuro-ophthalmic lesion noted in AIDS patients: Papilledema due to cryptococcal meningitis

1650. MC neuro-ophthalmologic manifestation of paralytic polio: Unilateral abducens nerve paresis

1651. MC isolated ocular motor nerve paresis that occurs in patients with AIDS: Abducens nerve paresis

1652. MC cause of ocular motor dysfunction in AIDS: HIV-associated dementia

1653. MC life-threatening mycosis in AIDS patients: Cryptococcosis

1654. MC neuro-ophthalmologic manifestation of sarcoidosis: Optic nerve dysfunction

1655. MC disorder of fixation associated with Multiple Sclerosis (MS): Nystagmus

1656. MC ocular motor nerve paresis that occurs in patients with MS: Abducens nerve paresis

1657. MC pupillary disturbance seen in patients with MS: Relative afferent pupillary defect (RAPD)

1658. MC presenting symptoms of Multiple Sclerosis (MS): Weakness, numbness, and paraesthesia of the extremities

1659. MC form of Encephalitis Lethargica (EL) (Von Economo Encephalitis): Somnolent-ophthalmoplegic type

1660. MC cause of ophthalmoparesis in Encephalitis Lethargica (EL):damage to the oculomotor nerve

1661. MC ocular sign during the acute stage of somnolent-ophthalmoplegic Encephalitis Lethargica: Ptosis

1662. MC ocular motor disturbance in Postencephalitis parkinsonism (PEP): Reduced or absent convergence

1663. MC ocular sign of Acute inflammatory demyelinating polyneuropathy (AIDP): Ophthalmoparesis

1664. MC affected nerve in Acute inflammatory demyelinating polyneuropathy (AIDP): Abducens nerve

1665. MC cause of acute generalized paralysis in the world: Acute inflammatory demyelinating polyneuropathy (AIDP)

1666. MC association of Foster–Kennedy syndrome: Meningiomas

1667. MC cause of supranuclear eyelid retraction: Lesions near the posterior commissure in the dorsal mesencephalon

1668. MC division of trigeminal nerve affected by trigeminal neuralgia (tic doulreux): Mandibular division

1669. MC site of spontaneous CSF leak:
   I. Area of the cribriform plate
   II. Well-pneumatized sphenoid sinus

1670. MC type of sphenoid sinus pneumatisation:
   I. Sellar (67%)
   II. Presellar (28%)
   III. Choncal (5%)

1671. MC neuro-ophthalmic sign found in primary familial systemic amyloidosis: Pupillary abnormalities

MOST COMMONS IN OPHTHALMOLOGY

1672. MC presenting symptoms of Lymphocytic hypophysitis (LH) or adenohypophysitis (autoimmune condition that occurs most frequently in women in the last trimester of pregnancy): Visual field defects and headache

1673. MC cause of Anton Syndrome: Bilateral occipital infarctions

1674. MC type of saccadic intrusions: Square-wave jerks (SWJs)

1675. MC neurologic manifestation of Takayasu's Arteritis: Syncope

1676. MC malformation of cortical development: Polymicrogyria

1677. MC neuro-ophthalmic manifestation of Diabetes mellitus: Diplopia

Ocular Pathology

General Pathology

1678. MC fixative used in frozen sections: 10% neutral buffered formalin

1679. MC indication of frozen section: To determine whether the resection margins are free of tumor

1680. MC stain used following microtome sectioning: Hematoxylin and eosin

1681. MC use of flow cytometry in clinical practice: Immunophenotyping hematopoietic proliferations

1682. MC granulomatous reactions seen in eye pathology:
   I. Tuberculosis
   II. Sarcoidosis
   III. Sympathetic ophthalmitis

1683. MC stain used to determine the type of bacterial infection: Giemsa stain

1684. MC ocular complication in Bone Marrow Transplant (BMT) patients:
   I. Keratoconjunctivitis sicca
   II. Cataract

1685. MC manifestation of Bone marrow suppression: Thrombocytopenia and hypersegmentation of neutrophils

1686. MC use of skin testing in ophthalmology: Diagnosis of tuberculosis

1687. MC method used to differentiate between local versus systemic origin of intraocular immunoglobulin: Goldmann-Witner coefficient (determined by comparison of the intraocular-fluid-to-serum ratio of virus-specific IgG to the intraocular-fluid-to-serum ratio of total IgG)

1688. MC used source of B lymphocytes for EBV cell culture: Umbilical cord lymphocytes

1689. MC histologic type of skin melanoma: Intraepidermal pagetoid (also known as superficial spreading)

1690. MC identified protein in KS tumor cells: LNA-1 (ORF-37)

1691. MC ocular manifestation of gout:

    I.   Red eyes (62%)

    II.   Pingueculae (25%)

    III.   Elevated IOP (14%)

    IV.   Asteroid hyalosis (4%)

1692. MC used tissue fixative: 10% neutral buffered formalin

Anterior Segment Pathology
1693. MC corneal dystrophy recurrence after keratoplasty:

MOST COMMONS IN OPHTHALMOLOGY

    I.   Reis Buckler Dystrophy

    II.   Granular

    III.   Lattice

    IV.   Macular

1694. MC cause of endothelium attenuation or absence in corneal specimen: Pseudophakic or aphakic bullous keratopathy

1695. MC systemic disorder associated with eye colobomas: CHARGE syndrome (coloboma of the retina/choroid, heart malformation, atresia choanae, genital hypoplasia, and ear malformation)

1696. MC cardiac abnormalities associated with CHARGE syndrome:

    I.   Atrial and ventricular septal defects

    II.   Patent ductus arteriosus (PDA)

    III.   Conotruncal heart defects and outflow anomalies

1697. MC disease studied from trabeculectomy specimens: Pigment Dispersion Syndrome (PDS)

1698. MC encountered iris abnormalities in clinical practice:

    I.   Nevus

    II.   Melanoma

    III.   Cysts

IV. Metastasis

1699. MC primary source to iris metastasis: Lung or breast carcinoma

1700. MC cause of brown stromal pigmentation in cornea specimens: Blood staining

1701. MC features seen in serial paraffin sections from well-preserved specimens in POAG: Hyalinisation and acellularity of the outer part of the trabecular meshwork

1702. MC specimen encountered in iridoschisis: From iridectomy taken in treatment of glaucoma

1703. MC finding in eyes enucleated in treatment of absolute glaucoma: Presence of closed angles with iridotrabecular and iridocorneal contact

1704. MC foreign body reaction encountered in conjunctiva: Stitch granuloma

1705. MC tumor of caruncle:
    I. Papilloma
    II. Nevus

1706. MC type of exogenous uveitis: Post traumatic iridocyclitis

1707. MC type of endogenous uveitis: Idiopathic inflammation (i.e., "garden-variety" anterior uveitis)

MOST COMMONS IN OPHTHALMOLOGY

1708. MC cause of rupture of Descemet's membrane (Haab's striae): Birth trauma

1709. MC eye involved in birth trauma causing Haab's striae: Left eye (because MC fetal presentation is left occiput anterior)

1710. MC ocular finding in Ehlers Danlos Syndrome: Marked epicanthal folds

1711. MC type of lesion in Erythema multiforme: Papules

1712. MC histopathologic finding in Conjunctivochalasis (CCh):
   I. Elastosis
   II. Chronic nongranulomatous inflammation

1713. MC inflammatory cell: Neutrophils

1714. MC type of cataract in Anterior Lenticonus: Nuclear cataract

1715. MC primary malignant neoplasm of the iris: Iris melanoma (5-8% of all uveal melanoma)

1716. MC part of iris involved in iridoschisis: Lower half of the iris

1717. MC types of HPV associated with conjunctival papilloma: HPV type 6 and 11

1718. MC subtype of conjunctival lymphoma: Extranodal marginal zone lymphoma (EMZL) of mucosa-associated lymphoid tissue (MALT)

1719. MC affected tissue by Ophthalmia Nodosa (immune reaction to caterpillar hairs): Conjunctiva

1720. MC congenital conjunctival lesion:

    I.   Dermoid

    II.   Dermolipoma

    III.   Ectopic lacrimal gland

    IV.   Osseous choristoma

1721. MC type of hamartoma (Greek word for "mistake mass") in conjunctiva: Capillary hemangioma

1722. MC cause of Papillary conjunctivitis (cobblestone arrangement of flattened nodules with central vascular cores):

    I.   Vernal and atopic keratoconjunctivitis

    II.   Response to a foreign body

1723. MC cause of Follicular conjunctivitis (small, dome-shaped nodules without a prominent central vessel):

    I.   Inflammation caused by pathogens such as viruses; atypical bacteria; toxins

    II.   Topical medications

1724. MC abnormality involving the lens epithelium: Posterior subcapsular cataract

1725. MC association of Sebaceous adenoma: Muir-Torre syndrome

1726. MC location of Iris hemangiomas: Inferior sector of the iris

1727. MC type of Iris hemangiomas: Iris arteriovenous malformations (AVM)

1728. MC complication of Iris arteriovenous malformations (AVM): Spontaneous hyphema

Posterior Segment Pathology

1729. MC genetically determined macular dystrophy: Stargardt-fundus flavimaculatus (S-FFM)

1730. MC juvenile macular dystrophies:
    I. X-linked juvenile retinoschisis
    II. Stargardt's disease
    III. Cone dystrophy
    IV. Vitelliform dystrophy

1731. MC primary ganglion cell disease:

MOST COMMONS IN OPHTHALMOLOGY

    I.   Kjer-type dominant optic atrophy (DOA)

    II.   Leber hereditary optic neuropathy (LHON)

1732. MC mutation in patients with LHON:

    I.   G11778A mutation (69%)

    II.   T14484C mutation (14%)

    III.   G3460Amutation (13%)

1733. MC mutation causing severe LHON phenotype:

    I.   A14495G

    II.   G11778A

1734. MC used immunostatin for melanoma (Neural crest markers):

    I.   A103 (Melan-A or Anti-MART-1)

    II.   S100 (anti-gp100)

    III.   HMB-45

    IV.   T311 (anti-tyrosinase)

1735. MC ocular pathology finding in congenital rubella syndrome: Salt and Pepper fundus

1736. MC systemic condition affecting uvea: Diabetes Mellitus

1737. MC systemic condition affecting retina: Diabetes Mellitus

MOST COMMONS IN OPHTHALMOLOGY

1738. MC anomaly caused by persistence of remnants of the primary vitreous or hyaloid vessel: Retention of fragments on the back of the lens (Mittendorf dot)

1739. MC entity involving the orbit in the group of Langerhans granulomatosis: Eosinophilic granuloma

1740. MC site of origin of medulloepithelioma (previously called diktyomas) in eye: Nonpigmented epithelium of the ciliary body

1741. MC presenting symptoms of medulloepithelioma: Pain and poor vision

1742. MC presenting signs of medulloepithelioma: Anterior chamber cyst or mass, leukocoria, and pupil abnormalities

1743. MC pseudogliomas:
  I. Persistent hyperplastic primary vitreous
  II. Retinal dysplasia
  III. Retinopathy of prematurity
  IV. Toxocara endophthalmitis
  V. Coats disease

1744. MC complicating granulomatous conditions following trauma:
  I. Sympathetic uveitis
  II. Phacoanaphylactic endophthalmitis

MOST COMMONS IN OPHTHALMOLOGY

    III.   Foreign body granulomas

1745. MC malformation of the peripheral fundus: Rosette (epiretinal epithelial proliferation in the configuration of warts or lappets) (clinically present in 27–30% and in autopsy eyes in 43%)

1746. MC tumor of most peripheral fundus: Malignant melanoma

1747. MC pathophysiology of retinal hole or tear: Secondary to degenerative disease in the retina and vitreous

1748. MC RPE cells change seen after detachment of neural retina: Cells become rounded and phagocytose lipoprotein (lipofuscin)

1749. MC location of cystic retinal tuft: Extrabasal or equatorial zone of retina

1750. MC location of noncystic retinal tuft: Inferior nasal quadrant, in anterior portion of the peripheral retina

1751. MC origin of retinal neovascularization:

    I.   Capillary bed at the edge of an infarcted area

    II.   Wall of a thickened venule

    III.   Wall of a hyalinised arteriole

1752. MC stain used to identify fungal elements in vitreous biopsy: PAS stain

1753. MC method of identification of toxoplasma in retinal specimens: Within cystic structures containing blue or purple dots (bradyzoites)

1754. MC location of bradyzoit cyst in toxoplasmosis retinal specimen: At the edge of the surviving retina

1755. MC location of lattice degeneration of retina:
   I. Adjacent to the superior and inferior vertical meridian
   II. Adjacent to the temporal horizontal meridian
   III. Adjacent to the nasal horizontal meridian

1756. MC quadrant of retina in which lattice degeneration is seen: Upper temporal quadrant

1757. MC location of Cobblestone degeneration (paving stone degeneration) in retina:
   I. Inferior temporal quadrant (~78%)
   II. Inferior nasal quadrant (~57%)

1758. MC location of retinal break in rhegmatogenous retinal detachment (RRD): Upper temporal quadrant

1759. MC pathophysiology of Coat's disease (Retinal Telangiectasia): Sectorial abnormality of the retinal vasculature

1760. MC quadrant involved by Coat's disease: Superior temporal quadrant

1761. MC precursor of disciform degeneration of macula: Exudative ARMD

1762. MC location of Myelinated Nerve Fibres (MNF): Area continuous with optic disc

1763. MC cause of focal interruption of axonal flow in the neural retinal nerve fiber layer that results in a cotton-wool spot: Ischemia

1764. MC type of Choroidal Neovascularisation (CNV):
    I.   Type 1: Sub RPE neovascularisation (More common)
    II.   Type 2: Sub Neural retina neovascularisation (Less common)

1765. MC type of macular lesion seen in Retinitis Pigmentosa:
    I.   Atrophy with RPE thinning (hypopigmentation) and mottled transmission on fluorescein angiography (58%)
    II.   Cystoid macular edema and leakage of fluorescein from foveal retinal capillaries (23%)
    III.   Cystic macular lesions with radial, inner neural retinal traction lines, often associated with epiretinal membranes that cause a surface wrinkling (19%)
    IV.   Perifoveal hyperautofluorescent ring representing abnormal accumulation of lipofuscin in the RPE

1766. MC cause of Posterior Vitreous Detachment (PVD):
    I.   Senescence

II. High myopia

III. Diabetes mellitus

IV. Ocular inflammation

V. Aphakia

1767. MC complaint of patient with PVD: Floaters

1768. MC location of Congenital hypertrophy of the RPE (CHRPE) lesions: Temporal fundus

1769. MC retinal layer involved in foveomacular retinoschisis: Inner nuclear layer

1770. MC developmental anomaly of the vitreous: Failure of the primary vitreous to completely regress (persistent hyperplastic primary vitreous PHPV)

1771. MC involved ocular site by Langerhans' cell histiocytosis: Choroid

1772. MC presentation of Langerhans' cell histiocytosis in the orbit: Lytic defect, usually affecting the superotemporal orbit or sphenoid wing and causing relapsing episodes of orbital inflammation, which are often initially misinterpreted as infectious orbital cellulitis

1773. MC type of cells seen in uveal nevi: Spindle A cells

1774. MC lymphoma that secondarily invade the uvea: High-grade large B-cell lymphoma

MOST COMMONS IN OPHTHALMOLOGY

1775. MC Non-Hodgkin lymphoma: High-grade large B-cell lymphoma

1776. MC type of calcinosis cutis occurring in eyelid: Subepidermal calcified nodule

1777. MC association of Necrobiotic xanthogranuloma (NXG): IgG monoclonal gammopathy

1778. MC ocular sign in Niemann-Pick syndrome: Macular cherry red spot

Orbital Pathology

1779. MC pathophysiology of Involutional ectropion: Ageing changes affecting the canthal tendons, the tarsus, the lid retractors and the orbicularis

1780. MC symptoms and signs indicating dysfunction of the lacrimal drainage system:

       I.   Epiphora

       II.   Punctal discharge

       III. Medial canthal swelling

1781. MC reason for enucleation in ophthalmology:

       I.   Painful blind eye with secondary glaucoma

       II.   Intraocular tumor suspected to be malignant and not amenable to (brachy and radiotherapy)

III. Avoidance of sympathetic ophthalmia after ocular trauma

1782. MC type of nevus cells found in nevus:
- I. Plump polyhedral nevus
- II. Slender spindle nevus cells
- III. Plump, fusiform, and dendritic
- IV. Balloon cells

1783. MC type of nevus:
- I. Intradermal nevus (MC with no malignant potential)
- II. Compound nevus (low malignant potential)
- III. Junctional nevus (low malignant potential)

1784. MC submitted specimen of Squamous Cell Carcinoma (SCC): Wide excision biopsy

1785. MC tissue source for hamartoma: Blood vessels and nerves

1786. MC clinical appearance of dermoid: Solid ovoid white mass (occasionally hair-bearing) at the limbus

1787. MC histopathologic type of meningioma seen within the orbit:
- I. Meningothelial (syncytial) meningioma
- II. Psammomatous meningioma

1788. MC mechanism of trans-scleral spread of choroidal melanoma: Scleral canals through which the ciliary arteries and nerves pass

1789. MC cells of origin in orbital lymphoma: B cell

1790. MC cells of origin in adnexal lymphoma: B cell

1791. MC primary orbital tumor producing exophthalmos: Cavernous hemangioma

1792. MC lesions simulating choroidal melanoma:

    I.   Choroidal nevus (49%)
    II. Peripheral haemorrhagic chorioretinopathy (8%)
    III. Congenital hypertrophy of the retinal pigment epithelium ((6%)
    IV. Haemorrhagic detachment of the retina or pigment epithelium (5%)
    V.   Circumscribed choroidal hemangioma (5%)
    VI. Age-related macular degeneration (4%)

1793. MC methods of optic nerve invasion by choroidal melanoma:

    I. By tumor extension from the neuroretina through the lamina cribrosa
    II. By direct extension into the optic nerve head between bruch's membrane and the border tissue of elschnig

MOST COMMONS IN OPHTHALMOLOGY

    III.   By direct invasion through the border tissue of elschnig

1794. MC clinical classification systems used for Retinoblastoma:

    I.   Reese–Ellsworth classification (REC)

    II.   International Classification (IC)

1795. MC route for retinoblastoma tumor to escape from the eye: Way of the optic nerve

1796. MC location of oncocytoma in eye: Caruncle

1797. MC hair follicle tumor: Pilomatrixoma (PM)

1798. MC peripheral nerve sheath tumor: Plexiform Neurofibroma

1799. MC ocular structure affected by IG4-Related Orbital Disease (IGRD): Lacrimal gland

1800. MC organ affected by Ig G4 related disease:

    I.   Pancreas

    II.   Hepatobiliary tract

    III.   Salivary glands

    IV.   Orbit

1801. MC acquired vascular lesion of eyelid: Pyogenic granuloma

1802. MC vascular tumor of the eyelid in children:

    I.   Capillary hemangioma

II. Lymphangioma

1803. MC vascular lesion of the orbit: Cavernous hemangioma

1804. MC type of leprosy in which ocular involvement is common: Lepromatous leprosy

1805. MC location of supernumerary punctum: Nasally to normal punctum

1806. MC subtype of Hodgkin's lymphoma in orbit: Nodular sclerosing variant

Ocular Pharmacology

General Ocular Pharmacology

1807. MC method used to administer treatments for ocular disease:

    I.   Topical drops (90%)

    II.   Ointments

1808. MC of all adverse reactions to topical medications: Toxic papillary keratoconjunctivitis

1809. MC pH value for biological fluids both inside and outside of cells: 7.4

1810. MC method of ocular drug delivery: Instillation of drops into the lower cul-de-sac

1811. MC sign of ocular toxicity from topical medication: Hyperemia

1812. MC herbicides/pesticides reported to cause ocular injury: Glyphosate

1813. MC isoforms of VEGFs:

    I.   VEGF 121

    II.   VEGF 165

    III. VEGF 189

1814. MC studied isoform of VEGF: VEGF-A 165

1815. MC class of agents prescribed as first-line therapy in the treatment of glaucoma: Prostaglandin analogues

1816. MC used first-generation cephalosporin for bacterial keratitis: Cefazolin

1817. MC used polyenes for treatment of fungal keratitis: Amphotericin B and natamycin

1818. MC used azoles for treatment of fungal keratitis:

    I.   Topical voriconazole

    II.   Oral ketoconazole and itraconazole

1819. MC preservative used in eye drops: Benzalkonium chloride(BAK) (it acts by interfering with the permeability of the bacterial cell membrane)

1820. MC used drug to treat Acanthamoeba keratitis: Topical propamidine isethionate

1821. MC non-pharmacological therapy for dry eye disease: Occlusion of the Tear Drainage System

1822. MC used route of administration to deliver drugs to the retina and vitreous: Intravitreal injection

1823. MC used agents for increasing viscosity of a topically applied ocular formulation:

    I.   Polyvinyl alcohol (PVA)

    II.   Derivatives of methylcellulose

1824. MC used nanoparticles for therapeutic purposes:

MOST COMMONS IN OPHTHALMOLOGY

    I.   Liposomes

    II.   Polymer drug conjugates

1825. MC sympathomimetic agents (α-adrenergic stimulant) used in ophthalmology for dilatation purposes: Phenylephrine

1826. MC used cardiac glycoside in laboratory: Ouabin

1827. MC used cardiac glycoside therapeutically: Digoxin

1828. MC studied intracellular modulator of aqueous humour secretion: Cyclic AMP

Adverse Effects

1829. MC side effect of topical gentamycin: SPK

1830. MC adverse ocular reaction: Curious visual disturbance, which includes brightly coloured appearances of objects as the main feature

1831. MC ocular side effect seen in patients on systemic sulpha drug therapy: Myopia

1832. MC ocular side effect of amphotericin B: Transient blurred vision

1833. MC systemic side effect of intravenous amphotericin B: Nephrotoxicity

1834. MC ocular side effect of voriconazole: Photopsia (enhanced visual perception, 'enhanced perception of light', 'brighter lights and objects', blurred or 'hazy' vision and photophobia 'dazzle' or 'glare')

1835. MC ocular side effect of Gabapentin: Decrease in central vision

1836. MC side effects due to carbamazepine: Transitory diplopia

1837. MC sign of clonidine overdose: Miosis

1838. MC ocular side effect of sildenafil:

    I. Transitory bluish discoloration of vision and impaired blue-green discrimination

    II. Hypersensitivity to light

    III. Minimal hazy vision

1839. MC adverse event of Periocular Botulinum injection:

    I. Ptosis

    II. Sicca

    III. Diplopia

1840. MC involved muscle in periocular Botox side effect: Inferior oblique

1841. MC systemic reactions of intravenous fluorescein angiographies: Nausea and vomiting

1842. MC ocular side effect of topical NSAIDs: Transitory irritation

MOST COMMONS IN OPHTHALMOLOGY

1843. MC side effect of oral NSAIDs: Gastrointestinal irritation

1844. MC ocular complication of corticosteroids: Cataract and secondary glaucoma

1845. MC ocular side effect of cyclopentolate: Transient stinging on instillation

1846. MC dose limiting toxicity of cyclophosphamide: Bone marrow depression

1847. MC secondary malignancy associated with cyclophosphamide:
    I. Acute myelocytic leukemia
    II. Bladder carcinoma

1848. MC side effect of azathioprine therapy:
    I. Leukopenia
    II. Thrombocytopenia
    III. Anemia

1849. MC reason for discontinuation of azathioprine therapy: Symptomatic GI discomfort

1850. MC side effect of leflunomide: Diarrhoea

1851. MC side effect of oral cyclosporine therapy:
    I. Nephrotoxicity
    II. Hypertension

1852. MC mode of Therapeutic drug monitoring for oral cyclosporine: Measuring a predose trough level approximately 12 hours after the last dose

1853. MC side effects of topical cyclosporine:
    I. Ocular burning sensation (14.7%)
    II. Stinging (4%)
    III. Conjunctival hyperemia (3.4%)

1854. MC side effect of sirolimus (rapamycin):
    I. Peripheral edema
    II. Hyperlipidaemia

1855. MC side effect of Adalimumab: Injection site reactions

1856. MC side effect of colchicine therapy: GI upset

1857. MC side effect of chlorambucil therapy: Dose dependant myelosuppression

1858. MC adverse event of Retisert implant: (at 3 years)
    I. Cataracts (93%)
    II. Elevated intraocular pressure requiring ocular antihypertensive medications (75%)
    III. The need for glaucoma surgery (40%)

MOST COMMONS IN OPHTHALMOLOGY

1859. MC side effect of IFN-alpha therapy:

    I.   Flu-like symptoms

    II.   Leukopenia

    III.   Alopecia

1860. MC used drugs for CMV retinitis: Ganciclovir, valganciclovir, foscarnet and cidofovir

1861. MC dose limiting side effect of ganciclovir therapy: Neutropenia (absolute neutrophil count < 1000/mm^3)

1862. MC mechanism of CMV resistance to ganciclovir:

    I.   Mutations in the UL97 gene encoding the viral phosphotransferase

    II.   DNA polymerase mutations (UL54 gene)

1863. MC major adverse effect associated with foscarnet administration: Nephrotoxicity causing Azotemia

1864. MC hematologic effect of foscarnet: Anemia

1865. MC ocular adverse effects of prostaglandin analogue:

    I.   Conjunctival hyperemia

    II.   Eyelash changes

    III.   Induced iris darkening

IV. Periocular skin pigmentation

1866. MC systemic adverse effects of prostaglandin analogue: Upper respiratory tract infection/cold/flu (4%)

1867. MC side effect of topical dorzolamide:

I. Stinging and burning upon instillation (33%)

II. Bitter taste (25%)

1868. MC side effect of topical brinzolamide: Blurring upon instillation (because it come as suspension)

1869. MC used miotic agent in glaucoma: Pilocarpine

1870. MC used cholinergic medication for glaucoma: Pilocarpine

1871. MC refractive change seen with pilocarpine: Induced myopia resulting from circular ciliary muscle contraction, zonular relaxation, and forward displacement of the lens with increased lens axial diameter

1872. MC encountered hazard after long-term pilocarpine instillation: Visual Blur

1873. MC prescribed hyperosmotic agent: Glycerol

1874. MC acute symptom/systemic side effects caused by apraclonidine: Dosage-dependent dry nose or mouth

1875. MC manifestation of glaucoma drug sensitivity: Dermatitis of the lid

1876. MC side effect of oral CAIs (Carbonic anhydrase inhibitors):

   Paraesthesias

1877. MC serious adverse event with oral CAIs: Aplastic anemia

1878. MC form of noncompliance to glaucoma therapy:
   I. Failure to take the medication
   II. Miss doses of medications

1879. MC adverse event associated with dapsone therapy:
   I. Dose-related hemolysis
   II. Methemoglobinemia

1880. MC rifabutin-induced uveitis type: Mild-to-moderate unilateral anterior uveitis with concomitant mild vitritis

1881. MC predisposing factor for uveitis associated with rifabutin: Persons also receiving fluconazole or a macrolide drug (which raises serum levels of rifabutin)

1882. MC indication for IFN- α in ophthalmology: Ocular involvement due to Behcet's disease (BD)

1883. MC side effect of mycophenolate mofetil: Gastrointestinal effects (31%)

1884. MC CNS side effect of cyclosporine: Tremors

1885. MC cause of Drug-induced linear IgA disease: Vancomycin

MOST COMMONS IN OPHTHALMOLOGY

1886. MC used topical anti-herpetic drugs on the market:

    I.   Acyclovir (ACV) ointment

    II.   Trifluorothymidine (TFT) drops

1887. MC side effect of oral acyclovir: Nausea, vomiting and abdominal pain

1888. MC mechanism of resistance to oral acyclovir:

    I.   Loss of synthesis of viral thymidine kinase so that acyclovir is not phosphorylated to its active form

    II.   Mutation causing thymidine kinase with altered substrate specificity that phosphorylates thymidine but not acyclovir

    III.   Mutation of the viral DNA polymerase gene induces a tered DNA polymerase that is not sensitive to inhibition by acyclovir triphosphate

1889. MC prescribed ocular antibiotic: Fluoroquinolones

1890. MC side effect of valacyclovir:

    I.   Headache

    II.   Nausea

    III.   Abdominal pain

    IV.   Dizziness

1891. MC side effect of ganciclovir:

MOST COMMONS IN OPHTHALMOLOGY

    I.   Blurred vision

    II.   Eye irritation

    III.   Punctate keratitis

    IV.   Conjunctival hyperemia

1892. MC drug inducing LABD (Linear IgA bullous dermatosis): Vancomycin

1893. MC medicines causing cornea verticiliata:

    I.   Amiodarone

    II.   Chloroquine and hydroxychloroquine

    III.   Indomethacin

    IV.   Phenothiazines

    V.   Vandetanib

1894. MC ocular side effect of amiodarone: Amiodarone-induced keratopathy (90%) (formation of verticillate, pigmented, corneal epithelial deposits)

1895. MC side effect of oral pilocarpine used for dry eye disease: Excessive sweating

1896. MC side effect of oral cevilemine used for dry eye disease:

    I.   Gastrointestinal symptoms (including nausea and diarrhoea)

    II.   Mild to moderate sweating

MOST COMMONS IN OPHTHALMOLOGY

1897. MC adverse event with alpha-2 adrenergic agonists (Apraclonidine and Brimonidine): Allergic blepharoconjunctivitis

1898. MC side effect of methotrexate administration:
    I. Aphthous stomatitis
    II. Nausea
    III. Diarrhoea
    IV. Elevation of hepatic transaminases
    V. Cytopenias

1899. MC drug-related conjunctival reaction: Nonspecific papillary reaction

1900. MC manifestation of cardiac glycoside toxicity:
    I. Frosted or snowy vision
    II. Xanthopsia (yellow-green vision)

1901. MC type of nystagmus seen during lithium therapy: Downbeat nystagmus

1902. MC side effect of capsaicin skin cream used for post-herpetic neuralgia: Transient burning of the skin

1903. MC corneal finding in toxic keratopathy due to topical ciprofloxacin: White crystalline precipitate (17% of treated eye)

MOST COMMONS IN OPHTHALMOLOGY

1904. MC systemic immunosuppression regimen in patients receiving ocular surface stem cell transplants: Combination of
    I.   Tacrolimus
    II. Mycophenolate mofetil
    III. Short course of oral prednisone

1905. MC drugs causing acute transitory myopia:
    I.   Diuretics
    II. Sulpha type drugs

1906. MC drug-related adverse events associated with omega 3 fatty acid supplementation: Dyspepsia and belching

1907. MC adverse event after instillation of ophthalmic solution of a selective ROCK inhibitor: Transient bulbar conjunctival hyperemia

1908. MC pathological finding in vagabatrin toxicity: Cone dysfunction

1909. MC side effects of pyridostigmine: Diarrhoea and cramping

1910. MC drug causing optic neuropathy: Ethambutol

1911. MC symptom of ethambutol related optic neuropathy: Blue-yellow colour changes

1912. MC used medical therapy for prolactinoma: Oral dopamine (D2) receptor agonists (bromocriptine, cabergoline, and quinagolide)

MOST COMMONS IN OPHTHALMOLOGY

1913. MC ocular symptoms during amiodarone treatment: Coloured halos around lights

1914. MC neurotoxicities associated with oral methotrexate:
   I. Acute or subacute encephalopathy
   II. Chronic progressive leukoencephalopathy
   III. Acute meningitis

1915. MC neurotoxicity associated with 5-FU: Subacute cerebellar syndrome

1916. MC neuro-ophthalmologic manifestation of 5-FU toxicity: Nystagmus

1917. MC neurotoxicity associated with systemic steroid use: Proximal myopathy

1918. MC ocular complication of systemic corticosteroids: Unilateral or bilateral posterior subcapsular cataracts

1919. MC chemotherapy regimen for retinoblastoma: Systemic three-agent chemotherapy with carboplatin, vincristine, and etoposide

1920. MC ocular side effects associated with intravitreal injection of methotrexate:
   I. Cataract
   II. Conjunctival hyperemia
   III. Transient keratopathy

1921. MC systemic adverse effects of anti-VEGFs:

   I. Hypertension

   II. Proteinuria

   III. Cardiovascular events

   IV. Bleeding associated with impaired wound healing

1922. MC used immunosuppressive agent for ocular Behcet's disease:

   Cyclosporin A (3–5 mg/kg/day)

1923. MC used steroid sparing immunosuppressant for myasthenia gravis:

   Azathioprine

1924. MC oral drug class used in blepharospasm:

   I. Anticholinergic-class drugs

   II. GABA-nergic drugs

1925. MC used somatostatin analogue in thyroid eye disease: Octreotide and lanreotide

1926. MC cause of iatrogenic punctal or canalicular stenosis: Ophthalmic medications

1927. MC chemotherapeutic agent causing canalicular stenosis:

   I. Docetaxel (Taxotere, administered to patients with metastatic breast carcinoma)

    II. 5-Flourouracil

1928. MC side effect of Intravenous Pamidronate sodium (Aredia): Bilateral anterior uveitis within the first 48 hours of drug exposure

1929. MC adverse effect of topical Ketorolac tromethamine: Stinging and burning on instillation (40%)

1930. MC adverse effect of Emedastine difumarate (0.05%, selective H1-receptor antagonist): Headache (11%)

1931. MC adverse effect of Iodoxamide (0.1%, mast cell stabilizer): Burning, stinging and discomfort upon instillation

1932. MC symptom complex associated with acetazolamide: Fatigue, anorexia, weight loss, malaise, depression and loss of libido

1933. MC ocular symptoms after the use of latanoprost:
    I. Foreign body sensation (13.3%)
    II. Stinging (9.3%)
    III. Itching and burning (7.5%)

1934. MC presentation of Topical Antiviral Toxicity: Diffuse punctate corneal epithelial erosions with conjunctival injection

1935. MC medications causing toxic follicular conjunctivitis: Atropine, antiviral agents, miotics, sulphonamides etc

Misc Ocular Pharmacology

1936. MC photochemical effect in use today: Photodynamic therapy (PDT)

1937. MC side effects from PDT with verteporfin: Photosensitivity and back pain

1938. MC used alkylating agent in cancer chemotherapy: Cyclophosphamide (Cytoxan)

1939. MC immunosuppressive used in children: Methotrexate

1940. MC used treatment regimen for Rosai-Dorfman disease: Combination of cyclophosphamide, vincristine, mercaptopurine, and prednisolone

1941. MC used treatment method for capillary hemangioma: Intralesional injection of steroids (40-80 mg of triamcinolone with 25 mg of methylprednisolone is directly injected into the lesion)

1942. MC used pharmacologic agent for Muller's muscle overaction in Thyroid eye disease: Alpha-adrenergic blocker guanethidine

1943. MC toxic cause of acute vertigo: Ethyl alcohol

1944. MC reason for giving premedication: To decrease anxiety

1945. MC used anxiolytic agents: Benzodiazepines

1946. MC reason for using anticholinergic medication as premedication: Prevention of reflex bradycardia

1947. MC used inhalational agent for induction of anaesthesia: Sevoflurane

1948. MC intravenous induction agent used for anaesthesia: Thiopental

1949. MC used drug to treat ocular hay fever: Topical antihistamines

1950. MC used systemic osmotic agent: Intravenous mannitol

1951. MC manifestation of corneal toxicity: Punctate epithelial keratopathy

1952. MC medications used to treat microsporidiosis in humans: Fumagillin and albendazole

Oculoplasty & Orbit

General Oculoplasty

1953. MC supernumerary muscles of orbit: Levator muscle of the trochlea (between the levator muscle of the superior eyelid and the trochlea)

1954. MC origin of Supraorbital artery: Ophthalmic artery on its medioptic part

1955. MC cause of Deep Superior Sulcus: Anophthalmia

1956. MC clinical manifestation of an orbital abnormality: Globe displacement

Eyelid

1957. MC cystic eyelid lesion: Epidermal inclusion cyst (Epidermoid cyst, Infundibular cyst)

1958. MC benign eyelid lesion:
  I. Squamous Papilloma (Acrocordon, Skin Tag, Fibroepithelial Polyp)
  II. Epidermal inclusion cysts
  III. Nevi

1959. MC benign eyelid tumor: Seborrhoeic Keratosis

MOST COMMONS IN OPHTHALMOLOGY

1960. MC benign tumors of the eyelid adnexa: Syringomata (benign tumors of the eccrine duct)

1961. MC eyelid involved by syringomas: Lower eyelid

1962. MC malignant tumor affecting periocular skin: Basal Cell Carcinoma

1963. MC eyelid lump in all ages: Meibomian Cysts (Chalazion)

1964. MC cause of chalazion: Blockage of a Meibomian gland

1965. MC complication of sling procedures in older patients: Development of dry eyes caused by iatrogenic lagophthalmos

1966. MC overlooked disease in patients referred with blepharoptosis: Myasthenia gravis

1967. MC cause of pseudoptosis: Contralateral upper lid retraction

1968. MC type of childhood ptosis: Myogenic ptosis

1969. MC type of myogenic ptosis: Congenital ptosis

1970. MC congenital lid abnormality: Congenital ptosis

1971. MC type of acquired ptosis: Aponeurotic ptosis (Levator dehiscence–disinsertion syndrome)

1972. MC pathology in aponeurotic blepharoptosis on ultrasound biomicroscopy: Thinned-out aponeurosis

MOST COMMONS IN OPHTHALMOLOGY

1973. MC causes of mechanical ptosis: Neoplastic or inflammatory infiltration or mass effect on the eyelid

1974. MC neuromuscular abnormality of the palpebral aperture: Ptosis

1975. MC causative mechanism of acquired ptosis: Dehiscence, disinsertion, or thinning of the levator aponeurosis

1976. MC etiology of levator dehiscence in younger and middle aged patients: Contact lens wear

1977. MC used procedure to correct blepharoptosis: Aponeurotic advancement

1978. MC performed Brow sling technique: Modifications of techniques by Wright and Crawford (that utilize two triangles of material to attach the eyelid at medial and lateral brow)

1979. MC type of entropion:
   I. Lower eyelid: Involutional entropion
   II. Upper eyelid: Cicatricial entropion

1980. MC cause of cicatricial entropion: Trachoma

1981. MC complication of entropion surgery: Recurrence

1982. MC cause of mechanical entropion: Neoplasm

1983. MC cause of Acute Spastic Entropion: Intraocular surgery in patients who had unrecognized or mild involutional eyelid changes preoperatively

1984. MC mechanism of congenital entropion: Defect in the lower lid posterior lamella leading to inverted eyelid margins

1985. MC form of ectropion:
   I.   Involutional ectropion
   II. Cicatricial ectropion

1986. MC cause of upper lid ectropion: Cicatricial ectropion

1987. MC reasons for recurrent ectropion following a surgical repair: Failure to recognize or address cicatricial eyelid changes

1988. MC eyelid malposition caused by eyelid burns: Cicatricial ectropion

1989. MC ocular complication if patients with Ichthyosis vulgaris: Ectropion

1990. MC cause of lid scarring:
   I.   Trauma
   II. Chalazia

1991. MC acquired vascular lesion of the eyelid: Pyogenic granuloma

1992. MC cause of pyogenic granuloma:
   I.   Post-trauma
   II. Post-surgery

1993. MC louse to infest the periocular region: Phthirus pubis

MOST COMMONS IN OPHTHALMOLOGY

1994. Mc symptom of infestation with Phthirus pubis: Intense pruritus associated with the injection of louse saliva into the skin during feeding

1995. MC location of upper eyelid coloboma: Junction of the inner third and the outer two thirds

1996. MC location of lower eyelid coloboma: Junction of the outer third and the inner two thirds

1997. MC syndromic cause of upper eyelid coloboma: Golderhar syndrome

1998. MC syndromic cause of lower eyelid coloboma: Treacher Collins syndrome

1999. MC dystonia associated with essential blepharospasm (EB): Oromandibular dystonia (This complex of EB and oromandibular dystonia is referred to as Meige's syndrome)

2000. MC form of eyelid neurofibroma: Plexiform neurofibroma

2001. MC type of cryptophthalmos: Complete cryptophthalmos

2002. MC syndromic cause of cryptophthalmos: Fraser syndrome

2003. MC eyelid condition that causes confusion when evaluating the patient with apparent ptosis: Dermatochalasis

2004. MC symptom of Symblepharon: Diplopia

2005. MC considerations to rule out when evaluating a child with suspected epiblepharon: Distichiasis and trichiasis

2006. MC eyelid involved by epiblepharon (horizontal fold of skin adjacent to eyelid margin): Lower eyelid

2007. MC performed procedure for epiblepharon: Excision of the skin fold and an underlying strip of orbicularis muscle

Lacrimal System

2008. MC location of fistula of lacrimal system: Under the medial canthal ligament

2009. MC infection of entire lacrimal apparatus: Dacryocystitis

2010. MC cause of acute dacryocystitis:
- I. Staphylococcus epidermidis
- II. Staphylococcus aureus

2011. MC recovered anaerobes from dacryocystitis:
- I. Peptostreptococcus
- II. Propionibacterium
- III. Prevotella
- IV. Fusobacterium

2012. MC organisms causing of congenital dacryocystitis:

　　I.　　Streptococcus pneumoniae

　　II.　　Staphylococcus

　　III.　　Gram-negative Enterobacteriaceae

2013. MC cause of dacryocanaliculitis:

　　I.　　Actinomyces israelii (filamentous gram-positive rod)

　　II.　　Nocardia and Streptomyces species

　　III.　　Propionibacterium propionicus

　　IV.　　Eikenella corrodens

2014. MC organism associated with bacterial dacryoadenitis: Staphylococcus aureus

2015. MC cause of viral dacryoadenitis:

　　I.　　Epstein Barr Virus

　　II.　　Mumps virus

2016. MC bacterial cause of chronic dacryoadenitis: Tuberculosis

2017. MC orbital manifestation of sarcoidosis: Chronic dacryoadenitis

2018. MC condition associated with alacrima: Familial dysautonomia or Riley–Day syndrome

2019. MC cause of NLDO (Naso-Lacrimal Duct Obstruction):

MOST COMMONS IN OPHTHALMOLOGY

    I.   Congenital: Membranous obstruction at the valve of Hasner

    II.   Young adult: Trauma or Dacryolith

    III.   Elderly >65 years: PANDO (primary acquired nasolacrimal duct obstruction)

2020. MC type of obstruction in Congenital NLDO:

    I.   Simple membranous obstruction of the distal valve of Hasner

    II.   Diffuse stenosis that extends along the distal nasolacrimal duct

2021. MC cause of Nasolacrimal sac infection:

    I.   Acute: β-hemolytic Streptococcus or Staphylococcus

    II.   Chronic: Streptococcus pneumoniae or Haemophilis influenza

2022. MC cause of chronic canaliculitis:

    I.   Actinomycosis

    II.   Fusobacterium

2023. MC involved canaliculus in chronic canaliculitis: Lower canaliculus

2024. MC presentation of Lacrimal gland tuberculosis: Nonspecific dacryoadenitis with or without abscess

2025. MC ocular manifestation of mumps: Dacryoadenitis

2026. MC cause of internal mechanical obstruction of nasolacrimal system: Dacryoliths

2027. MC location of dacryolith: Lacrimal sac

2028. MC cause of a watering eye (epiphora): Blocked nasolacrimal duct

2029. MC cause of epiphora in children: Congenital nasolacrimal duct obstruction (CNLDO)

2030. MC location of obstruction in congenital NLDO: Obstruction is at the opening of the nasolacrimal system due to an imperforate valve of Hasner

2031. MC location of canalicular stenosis: Membranous stenosis at the internal punctum

2032. MC site of block in Adult NLDO: Junction of the sac and the nasolacrimal duct

2033. MC site of block in Infant with NLDO: Lower portion of the nasolacrimal duct

2034. MC cause of lacrimal dysfunction: Age related lacrimal degeneration

2035. MC situations in which lacrimal pump failure is present despite patency of the membranous lacrimal conduit: Facial nerve paresis

2036. MC origin of Lacrimal ductal cyst: Palpebral lobe of lacrimal gland

2037. Mc location of Ectopic lacrimal gland:
   I. Eyelid

II. Conjunctiva

2038. MC treatment of Non patent Nasolacrimal drainage system: Probing

2039. MC used canalicular bypass tube: Lester Jones' Pyrex tube

2040. MC anatomical site for Dacryops:

    I. Lacrimal gland (Simple dacryops)

    II. Accessory lacrimal gland

    III. Ectopic lacrimal tissue

2041. MC implied etiology for Dacryops: Trachoma

Orbit

2042. MC non-infectious orbital disease:

    I. Thyroid related ophthalmopathy (Graves' ophthalmopathy)

    II. Lymphoproliferative disease

    III. Idiopathic orbital inflammatory syndrome (IOIS)

2043. MC painful orbital disease in adults: Idiopathic orbital inflammatory syndrome (IOIS)

2044. MC cause of unilateral or bilateral proptosis: Thyrotoxicosis

MOST COMMONS IN OPHTHALMOLOGY

2045. MC intraorbital parasitic infection:

   I.   Cysticercosis

   II. Hydatid cyst (Echinococcus granulosus)

2046. MC helminthic ocular infection: Cysticercosis

2047. MC presentation of orbital hydatidosis: Proptosis

2048. MC cause of unilateral proptosis in adults:

   I.   Thyroid associated ophthalmopathy

   II. Lymphoproliferative disorders

   III. Idiopathic orbital inflammation

2049. MC cause of unilateral proptosis in children:

   I.   Dermoid cyst

   II. Hemangiomas

2050. MC finding in grave's ophthalmopathy: Eyelid retraction

2051. MC cause of lagophthalmos: Orbicularis oculi paralysis due to seventh-nerve dysfunction

2052. MC location of subcutaneous periorbital dermoid cyst:

   I.   Lateral brow (superotemporal quadrant of orbital rim)

   II. Upper lid adjacent to the frontozygomatic suture (superonasal quadrant of rim)

MOST COMMONS IN OPHTHALMOLOGY

2053. MC location of Phakomatous choristoma: Inferonasal aspect of the lower eyelid

2054. MC tumor of infancy: Capillary hemangioma (10% of infants)

2055. MC benign periorbital tumor of childhood: Capillary hemangioma ('strawberry nevus')

2056. MC visceral vascular malformation associated with adnexal capillary hemangioma: Laryngeal hemangioma (29%)

2057. MC benign primary orbital tumor of adults: Cavernous hemangioma

2058. MC malignant primary orbital tumor of adults: Orbital lymphoma

2059. MC site of orbital lymphoma: Lacrimal fossa

2060. MC orbital lesion in immunocompromised AIDS population: Lymphoma

2061. MC involved extraocular muscles in orbital lymphoma: Superior rectus - levator complex

2062. MC ocular structure involved by lymphomatous disease of the orbit: Lacrimal gland

2063. MC used classification for lymphoma: Revised European-American Lymphoma (REAL) classification

2064. MC subtype of orbital lymphoma: Marginal zone B-cell lymphoma (MALT-lymphomas)

MOST COMMONS IN OPHTHALMOLOGY

2065. MC vascular tumor of the orbit: Cavernous hemangiomas

2066. MC cause of progressive visual disturbance in patients with cavernous hemangioma: Vitreous haemorrhage

2067. MC surgical approach for cavernous hemangioma:
   I.   Intraconal lesion: Lateral orbitotomy
   II. Extraconal lesion: Anterior orbital approach

2068. MC orbital tumor in adults: Metastatic tumor

2069. MC entrapped muscle in orbital floor fracture: Inferior rectus

2070. MC cause of enophthalmos: Orbital blowout fracture

2071. MC cause of restrictive strabismus in patients with posttraumatic enophthalmos: Entrapment of the extraocular muscles within the fracture

2072. MC carcinoma causing enophthalmos: Metastatic sclerosing carcinoma of the breast

2073. MC feature of idiopathic orbital inflammation: Pain

2074. MC form of Idiopathic Orbital Inflammatory Syndrome (IOIS) to affect children: Posterior scleritis

2075. MC orbital structure involved in Idiopathic Orbital Inflammatory Syndrome (IOIS): Lacrimal gland

2076. MC extraocular muscle involved by Idiopathic Orbital Inflammatory Syndrome (IOIS):
- I. Superior muscle group (levator and superior rectus)
- II. Medial rectus

2077. MC symptom in adult Idiopathic Orbital Inflammatory Syndrome (IOIS):
Pain

2078. MC sign in adult Idiopathic Orbital Inflammatory Syndrome (IOIS):
Periorbital edema/swelling

2079. MC locations for intracranial extension of Idiopathic Orbital Inflammatory Syndrome (IOIS):
- I. Cavernous sinus
- II. Middle cranial fossa

2080. MC orbital processes that present with similar clinical pictures as Idiopathic Orbital Inflammatory Syndrome (IOIS):
- I. Thyroid eye disease
- II. Orbital cellulitis

2081. MC cause of infectious orbital myositis:
- I. Staphylococcus aureus
- II. Streptococcus pyogenes

III. Clostridium welchii

2082. MC cause of globe pulsation: Acquired carotid-cavernous fistulas

2083. MC peripheral nerve tumors of the orbit:

    I. Schwannomas

    II. Neurofibromas

2084. MC pathway for odontico-orbital infections: Through the paranasal sinuses

2085. MC extraocular muscle involved in Congenital orbital fibrosis (one of syndrome causing myogenic congenital ptosis): Inferior rectus

2086. MC orbital infection seen in association with HIV/AIDS: Invasive aspergillosis

2087. MC lesion of intraconal space causing axial proptosis:

    I. Cavernous hemangioma

    II. Schwannoma

    III. Neurofibroma

2088. MC intraconal cystic lesion: Hydatid cyst

2089. MC fungal disease involving orbit:

    I. Phycomycosis (aka Mucormycosis)

    II. Aspergillosis

2090. MC underlying disorder in Mucormycosis:

    I.   Diabetes Mellitus with Ketoacidosis

    II.   Severe immunosuppression

2091. MC genera isolated in orbital Phycomycosis:

    I.   Rhizopus

    II.   Mucor

    III.   Absidia

2092. MC vasculitis that involve the orbit:

    I.   Wegener's granulomatosis

    II.   Polyarteritis nodosa

2093. MC site of orbital meningocele: Inner angle of the orbit or at the root of the nose

2094. MC cause of eyelid pulsations: Neurofibromatosis (due to absence of sphenoid bone which allows brain pulsations to be transmitted to the orbital contents)

2095. MC arteriovenous malformation affecting the orbit: Carotid cavernous sinus fistula (CSF)

2096. MC cause of orbital pain: Referred pain

2097. MC cause of referred orbital pain: Tension headache

2098. MC cause of orbital dystopia: Congenital anomalies of orbital development (like craniosynostosis, hemifacial microsomia, and orbitofacial clefts)

2099. MC muscle involved in monomuscular myositis:

    I.   Medial rectus

    II.   Lateral rectus

2100. MC nonaxial type of globe displacement: Hypo-ophthalmos (downward displacement of the globe) associated with disruption of the orbital floor

2101. MC used synthetic orbital implants:

    I.   Silicone sphere

    II.   Hydroxyapatite sphere

    III.   Porous polyethylene

2102. MC complication of Hydroxyapatite (HA) orbital implants: Implant exposure

2103. MC presenting sign of venous-lymphatic malformation of orbit: Painful unilateral proptosis resulting from spontaneous haemorrhage

Orbital Cellulitis

2104. MC cause of orbital cellulitis:

    I.   Ethmoidal sinusitis

MOST COMMONS IN OPHTHALMOLOGY

    II.   Frontal sinusitis

    III.   Sphenoid sinusitis

2105. MC cause of orbital cellulitis in young children: H. influenza

2106. MC organisms causing orbital cellulitis:

    I.   S. aureus

    II.   Streptococci

2107. MC cause of orbital cellulitis in children: Streptococcus

2108. MC cause of proptosis in children:

    I.   Orbital cellulitis

    II.   Thyroid Associated Orbitopathy

2109. MC cause of painful rapidly progressive proptosis: Orbital cellulitis

2110. MC location of subperiosteal abscess in orbital cellulitis: Medial orbital wall (since the medial orbital wall adjacent to the ethmoid sinus is the thinnest of all the orbital walls)

2111. MC orbital disease in children over 3 years: Preseptal cellulitis

2112. MC cause of preseptal cellulitis: Contiguous infection of the soft tissues of the face and eyelids secondary to local trauma, foreign bodies or insect or animal bites

2113. MC microorganism causing preseptal cellulitis:

MOST COMMONS IN OPHTHALMOLOGY

    I.   Streptococcus pneumoniae

    II.   Staphylococcus aureus

    III.   Other Streptococcus species

    IV.   Anaerobes

2114. MC pathogen in patients with preseptal cellulitis from trauma:

Staphylococcus aureus

2115. MC organism causing Necrotizing fasciitis: Group A beta-hemolytic streptococcus

Thyroid Eye Disease (TED)

2116. MC cause of unilateral exophthalmos: Grave's ophthalmopathy

2117. MC cause of bilateral exophthalmos: Grave's ophthalmopathy

2118. MC cause of lagophthalmos associated with proptosis: Thyroid ophthalmopathy

2119. MC ocular symptom when TED is first confirmed: Dull, deep orbital pain or discomfort (which affects 30% of patients)

2120. MC cause of upper lid retraction:

    I.   Thyroid eye disease

    II.   Dorsal midbrain syndrome (collier sign)

III. Contralateral ptosis

2121. MC cause of Supranuclear bilateral eyelid retraction (Collier sign):

Lesions of the dorsal mesencephalon

2122. MC cause of lower lid retraction: Thyroid ophthalmopathy

2123. MC ocular sign of thyroid eye disease:
- I. Upper lid retraction (Dalrymple sign)
- II. Lid lag

2124. MC identified dilated vessels on echography in thyroid associated ophthalmopathy:
- I. Medial collateral vein
- II. Superior ophthalmic vein

2125. MC abnormality of the optic nerve seen in thyroid ophthalmopathy: Papilledema

2126. MC CT scan finding in thyroid ophthalmopathy: Enlargement of the extraocular muscles with relative sparing of the tendinous insertion

2127. MC muscle involved in thyroid eye disease (Graves' Ophthalmopathy):
- I. Inferior rectus
- II. Medial rectus

2128. MC enlarged muscles as detected by echography in Thyroid Associated Orbitopathy (TAO): Superior rectus–levator complex

2129. MC surgery performed for Thyroid Associated Orbitopathy (TAO): Removal of the orbital floor and medial wall

2130. MC misalignment seen in Thyroid Associated Orbitopathy (TAO): Combined esotropia and hypertropia

2131. MC extraocular muscle (EOM) limitation in Thyroid Associated Orbitopathy (TAO): Impaired upward gaze

2132. MC cause of blindness secondary to thyroid orbitopathy: Optic neuropathy

2133. MC form of extraocular muscle surgery performed for thyroid ophthalmopathy: Recession of tight fibrous inferior rectus muscle

2134. MC upper lid disorder requiring surgical therapy in patients with Thyroid Associated Orbitopathy (TAO): Upper lid retraction due to levator muscle fibrosis

2135. MC used method of elevating the lid in Thyroid Associated Orbitopathy (TAO): Recessing the lower lid retractors by placing a tissue spacer between the inferior margin of the inferior tarsus and the lower lid retractor

2136. MC extrathyroidal expression of Graves' disease: Graves' orbitopathy (GO)

2137. MC orbital disorder: Graves' congestive orbitopathy

2138. MC cause of single or multiple extraocular muscle thickening: Graves' disease

2139. MC cause of extraocular muscle enlargement: TRO (Thyroid Related Orbitopathy)

2140. MC specific inflammation of the orbit: TRO

2141. MC diseases mimicking Graves' Orbitopathy (GO):
    I. Orbital meningioma
    II. Orbital myositis
    III. Caroticocavernous fistula
    IV. Non-Hodgkin lymphoma

Misc Oculoplasty

2142. MC cause of External ophthalmomyiasis: Sheep botfly Oestrus ovis

2143. MC location of fly larvae in ophthalmomyiasis: Conjunctiva

2144. MC complication during enucleation procedure: Bleeding

2145. MC association of Floppy eyelid syndrome: Obstructive sleep apnea

2146. MC type of sleep apnea:

   I. Obstructive

   II. Central

   III. Mixed

2147. MC ophthalmic treatment for facial palsy: Use of frequent lubricants

2148. MC cause of acute facial palsy: Bell's palsy

2149. MC mechanism of Aberrant Facial Nerve Regeneration:

   I. Wallerian degeneration of axons with resultant abnormal branching during axonal regeneration

   II. Nuclear hyperexcitability

   III. Central cortex reorganization

2150. MC source of hydroxyapatite sphere material: Sea coral

2151. MC used wrapping material for hydroxyapatite sphere implant: Donor sclera

2152. MC socket problem causing discharge: Dryness and decreased tear production

2153. MC eyelid problem leading to socket discharge: Giant papillary conjunctivitis (GPC)

2154. MC complications associated with evisceration: Exposure and extrusion of the implant

2155. MC used graft for fornix reconstruction: Labial or buccal mucous membrane

2156. MC pathogenesis of orbital tuberculosis: Haematogenous spread from a pulmonary focus

Oncology

General Eye Oncology

2157. MC intraocular tumor of adults: Uveal naevi (5% of population)

2158. MC malignant intraocular tumor of adults: Choroidal Metastases (2 to 9% patients with known cancer)

2159. MC primary intraocular malignancy in adults: Uveal Melanoma (0.7/100,000 per year)

2160. MC primary tumor for choroidal metastases:

   I. Breast cancer (47-60%)

   II. Lung cancer (21%)

   III. Gastrointestinal tract (4%)

   IV. Kidney (2%)

   V. Skin (2%)

   VI. Prostate (2%)

2161. MC primary tumor for choroidal metastases in Male: Lung Ca

2162. MC primary tumor for choroidal metastases in Female:

   I. Breast Carcinoma (70-80%)

   II. Lung carcinoma (10%)

2163. MC site of ocular metastasis:

MOST COMMONS IN OPHTHALMOLOGY

I. Posterior uvea/choroid (MC in adults)

II. Orbit (MC in children)

III. Iris

IV. Ciliary body

2164. MC site of ocular metastasis in children: Orbit

2165. MC primary intraocular malignancy of childhood:

I. Retinoblastoma (1 in 15000 to 1 in 18000 live births)

II. Embryonal Medulloepithelioma

2166. MC primary cancer for ocular metastasis:

I. Breast

II. Lung

III. Unknown

2167. MC technique to acquire intraocular tissue: Fine-needle aspiration biopsy (FNAB)

2168. MC indication for choroidal tumor biopsy: To determine the site of the primary malignancy in a patient with an unequivocal metastasis

Anterior Segment Oncology
2169. MC epibulbar tumors in children: Epibulbar choristomas

2170. MC malignancy of the conjunctiva in the United States: Conjunctival SCC

2171. MC location of Conjunctival SCC: Bulbar conjunctiva in the interpalpebral zone

2172. MC ocular surface neoplasm: Conjunctival Intraepithelial Neoplasia (CIN) (Now broadly classified as OSSN – Ocular Surface Squamous Neoplasia)

2173. MC presenting symptom of Conjunctival Intraepithelial Neoplasia (CIN):
   I. Red eye (68%)
   II. Ocular irritation (57%)

2174. MC malignancy seen in patients of AIDS:
   I. Kaposi's sarcoma
   II. High-grade B-cell non-Hodgkin lymphoma

2175. MC neoplasm to affect the CNS in AIDS patients: High-grade B-cell non-Hodgkin lymphoma

2176. MC conjunctival tumor associated with AIDS: SCC

2177. MC systemic condition associated with Kaposi's sarcoma: AIDS

2178. MC presentation of Kaposi's sarcoma:
   I. Eyelid tumor

II. Conjunctival tumor

2179. MC location of conjunctival Kaposi's sarcoma:

   I. Lower fornix

   II. Bulbar conjunctiva

   III. Upper fornix

2180. MC approach to detect microscopic metastases: Technetium-labelled sulphur colloid and blue dye

2181. MC used radioactive material for OSSN Brachytherapy:

   I. Strontium-90

   II. Ruthenium-106

2182. MC site for PAM: At the limbus and epibulbar interpalpebral region

2183. MC form of systemic amyloidosis: Light chain amyloidosis

2184. MC location of iris melanocytoma: Inferior quadrant of iris

2185. MC lesion to be confused with iris melanoma: Primary cyst of the iris

2186. MC malignancy of Iris: Metastasis from Lung cancer

2187. MC nonpigmented ocular surface tumor: OSSN (Ocular surface squamous neoplasia)

2188. MC misdiagnosis of OSSN:

   I. Pinguecula

MOST COMMONS IN OPHTHALMOLOGY

II. Pterygium

III. Actinic keratosis

IV. Squamous papilloma

V. Episcleritis

2189. MC melanocytic tumor of the conjunctiva: Conjunctival melanocytic nevus

2190. MC conjunctival tumor: Conjunctival melanocytic nevus

2191. MC location of Conjunctival melanocytic nevus:

I. Bulbar conjunctiva

II. Caruncle

III. Plica semiluminaris

2192. MC location of conjunctival melanoma:

I. Bulbar conjunctiva

II. Limbus

III. Palpebral conjunctiva is rarely involved

2193. MC local lymph nodes involved in conjunctival melanoma:

I. Preauricular

II. Submandibular

III. Deeper cervical lymph nodes

MOST COMMONS IN OPHTHALMOLOGY

2194. MC sites of distant metastasis in conjunctival melanoma:

   I.   Brain

   II. Liver

   III. Lung

2195. MC premalignant lesion of conjunctival melanoma: Primary acquired melanosis (PAM) with atypia

2196. MC lymphoproliferative conjunctival lesion: Non-Hodgkin lymphoma (NHL) of B-cell origin

2197. MC lymphoma to affect the conjunctiva: Extranodal marginal zone lymphoma of the mucosa-associated lymphoid tissue (MALT)

2198. MC presentation of conjunctival lymphoma: Salmon patch (diffuse, slightly elevated, pink, fleshy mass)

2199. MC location of conjunctival lymphoma: Forniceal or midbulbar conjunctiva, hidden under the eyelid in the superior and inferior quadrants

2200. MC reported primary cancers associated with conjunctival metastasis:

   I.   Breast

   II. Lung

   III. Cutaneous melanoma

MOST COMMONS IN OPHTHALMOLOGY

2201. MC primary neoplasm of cornea: Squamous cell carcinoma

2202. MC site of metastasis of Malignant melanoma of the conjunctiva and cornea:
   I. Ipsilateral facial lymph nodes
   II. Brain
   III. Lung
   IV. Liver

Eyelid Oncology

2203. MC Human malignancy: Skin cancer (MC is BCC)

2204. MC skin cancer of the eyelid:
   I. BCC (Basal Cell Carcinoma)
   II. SCC (Sebaceous Cell Carcinoma)
   III. SGC (Sebaceous Gland Carcinoma)
   IV. MM (Malignant melanoma)

2205. MC clinical presentation of BCC: Well-circumscribed nodular lesion with pearly edges and some telangiectasia with or without ulceration

2206. MC site of periocular BCC:
   I. Lower lid (50-60%)

MOST COMMONS IN OPHTHALMOLOGY

    II.   Medial canthus (25-30%)

    III.   Upper lid (15%)

    IV.   Lateral canthus (5%)

2207. MC site of BCC metastasis: Lymph nodes

2208. MC type of BCC:

    I.   Nodular/ulcerative (75%)

    II.   Morphea/sclerosing

    III.   Superficial

    IV.   Basosquamous

2209. MC site of periocular SCC:

    I.   Lower eyelid (51%)

    II.   Medial canthus (36%)

    III.   Upper eyelid (23%)

    IV.   Lateral canthus

2210. MC conditions mistaken for SCC:

    I.   Inverted follicular keratosis

    II.   Benign keratosis

    III.   Keratoacanthoma

    IV.   Pseudoepitheliomatous hyperplasia

MOST COMMONS IN OPHTHALMOLOGY

    V.   Basal cell carcinoma

2211. MC risk factors for SCC:

    I.   Exposure to ultraviolet light

    II.   Fair complexion

2212. MC pattern of SGC (Sebaceous Gland Carcinoma): Lobular

2213. MC location of periocular SGC:

    I.   Upper lid

    II.   Lower lid

    III.   Caruncle

    IV.   Brow

2214. MC presentation of SGC: Asymptomatic round subcutaneous yellowish nodule in the periocular region most often on the upper eyelid

2215. MC path of metastasis of eyelid SGC: Via the lymphatic channels to regional lymph nodes

2216. MC site of metastasis from SGC upper lid:

    I.   Preauricular

    II.   Parotid

2217. MC site of metastasis from SGC lower lid:

    I.   Submandibular

II. Cervical

2218. MC clinical variant of SGC:

    I. Solitary nodule of the eyelid

    II. Diffuse thickening of the eyelid

2219. MC glands from which SGC origins:

    I. Meibomian glands

    II. Zeis' glands

    III. sebaceous glands in the caruncle

2220. MC variant of cutaneous melanoma:

    I. Superficial spreading melanoma (70%)

    II. Nodular melanoma (16%)

    III. Acral lentiginous melanoma (9%)

    IV. Lentigo maligna melanoma (5%)

2221. MC type of melanoma affecting eyelid:

    I. Lentigo maligna melanomas

    II. Superficial spreading melanoma

    III. Nodular melanomas

2222. MC presentation of patients with periocular melanoma: Morphologic change in a preexisting pigmented lesion

MOST COMMONS IN OPHTHALMOLOGY

2223. MC location of periocular melanoma:

  I. Lower eyelid

  II. Upper lid

  III. Lateral canthus

  IV. Medial canthus

2224. MC adverse effects to occur after radiotherapy: Acute loss of eyelashes

2225. MC benign epithelial tumor of eyelid: Squamous papilloma

2226. MC pigmented eyelid lesion: Nevi

2227. MC location of nevi of eyelid: Along the eyelid border

2228. MC pigmented eyelid malignancy: Pigmented BCC

2229. MC site of involvement in Merkel cell tumor: Upper lid

2230. MC primary tumor that metastasize to eyelid: Adenocarcinoma of the breast

2231. MC sweat gland carcinoma of the eyelid: Mucin-secreting adenocarcinoma

2232. MC precancerous cutaneous lesion: Actinic keratosis (AK)

2233. MC treatment modality used for eradicating Actinic Keratosis: Destruction via Cryosurgery

2234. MC vascular tumor in children: Infantile capillary hemangioma

2235. MC ocular complication of adnexal capillary hemangiomas: Visual loss resulting from amblyopia

2236. MC type of retention cyst in eyelid: Sudoriferous cyst (originating from sweat gland)

2237. MC location of malignant syringoma (sweat gland adenocarcinoma): Nasolabial and periorbital regions

2238. MC cutaneous feature of organoid nevus syndrome: Sebaceous nevus of Jadassohn

2239. MC soft tissue tumor of infancy: Infantile hemangiomas

2240. MC complication of hemangiomas: Ulceration

2241. MC complication of periocular hemangioma: Compression of the globe leading to a deformed cornea and resulting in astigmatism

2242. MC cutaneous xanthoma: Eyelid Xanthelasma (xanthelasma palpebrarum)

2243. MC inherited disorder leading to hypomelanosis: Oculocutaneous albinism

2244. MC benign lesions of the eyelid: Squamous cell papilloma

Orbital Oncology

2245. MC location for orbital metastasis:

    I.   Lateral orbit 39%

    II.   Superior orbit 32%

    III.   Medial orbit 20%

    IV.   Inferior orbit 12%

2246. MC cause of bilateral orbital and sino-orbital disease: Breast carcinoma

2247. MC benign congenital tumor in children: Dermoid cyst

2248. MC tumor to metastasize to the orbit in adult:

    I.   Breast

    II.   Lung

    III.   Prostate

    IV.   Skin melanoma

2249. MC cystic lesion of orbit:

    I.   Dermoid Cyst (62%)

    II.   Mucocele (20%)

    III.   Epithelial cyst (8%)

    IV.   Lacrimal gland cysts (5%)

    V.   Microphthalmos with cyst (2%)

- VI. Colobomatous cyst (<1%)
- VII. Parasitic cyst (<1%)
- VIII. Hematic cyst (<1%)

2250. MC neurogenic orbital tumors:
- I. Sphenoid wing meningioma (30%)
- II. Optic nerve glioma (22%) (It is MC neurogenic in paediatric population)
- III. Neurofibroma (19%)
- IV. Optic sheath meningioma (11%)
- V. Schwannoma (9%)
- VI. Other (4%)
- VII. Carcinoid tumor (<1%)
- VIII. Malignant peripheral nerve tumor (<1%)
- IX. Neuroblastoma (<1%)

2251. MC mesenchymal orbital tumors:
- I. Dermolipoma (44%)
- II. Rhabdomyosarcoma (22%) (MC malignant mesenchymal tumor of children)
- III. Fibrous histiocytoma (20%)

MOST COMMONS IN OPHTHALMOLOGY

    IV.   Liposarcoma (4%)

    V.   Fibrosarcoma (3%)

    VI.   Leiomyosarcoma (<1%)

    VII.   Juvenile xanthogranuloma (<1%)

    VIII.   Lipoblastomatosis (<1%)

    IX.   Lipoma (<1%)

2252. MC orbital vascular lesions:

    I.   Cavernous hemangioma (26%)

    II.   Capillary hemangioma (24%)

    III.   Lymphangioma (17%)

    IV.   Orbital varices (13%)

    V.   AV shunt (13%)

    VI.   Hemangiopericytoma (1%)

2253. MC orbital bone tumors:

    I.   Osteoma (39%)

    II.   Ewing's sarcoma (14%)

    III.   Aneurysmal bone cyst (11%)

    IV.   Ossifying fibroma (11%)

    V.   Fibrous dysplasia (7%)

VI.   Osteosarcoma (7%)

   VII. Brown tumor (7%)

   VIII. Chondrosarcoma (4%)

2254. MC location of fibrous histiocytoma of orbit: Superonasal orbital quadrant

2255. MC soft tissue sarcoma in adults: Liposarcoma

2256. MC neoplasm of lacrimal sac:
   I. Epithelial tumors
   II. Lymphoid tumors

2257. MC malignant epithelial tumors of lacrimal sac:
   I. squamous cell carcinoma (50% rate of recurrence)
   II. Transitional cell carcinoma (100% mortality)

2258. MC site of metastasis of SCC of lacrimal sac:
   I. Lung
   II. Bone

2259. MC benign epithelial tumors of lacrimal sac: Squamous cell papilloma

2260. MC nonepithelial tumor of lacrimal sac: Lymphomas or reticulcses (50% all nonepithelial tumors)

2261. MC lacrimal sac swelling: Lacrimal sac mucocele

MOST COMMONS IN OPHTHALMOLOGY

2262. MC vascular tumor of lacrimal sac: Hemangiopericytoma

2263. MC mode of spread of lacrimal sac tumors: Direct extension

2264. MC maxillary sinus tumors: Squamous cell carcinomas

2265. MC primary bone malignant tumor: Osteosarcoma

2266. MC location of NSOI (Non Specific Orbital Inflammation):
    I. Extraocular muscles
    II. Lacrimal glands
    III. Anterior
    IV. Apical (orbital apex)
    V. Diffuse orbital inflammation

2267. MC mesenchymal orbital tumor in adults: Fibrous histiocytoma

2268. MC bony tumors of the orbit: Primary Osteoma

2269. MC site of origin of osteoma: Frontal sinus

2270. MC location of Aneurysmal Bone Cyst of Orbit: Orbital Roof

2271. MC CT scan pattern of optic nerve sheath meningiomas: Diffuse tubular enlargement

2272. MC symptom of optic nerve sheath meningioma: Loss of vision

2273. MC Benign tumor of lacrimal gland: Pleomorphic adenoma (Benign mixed tumor)

MOST COMMONS IN OPHTHALMOLOGY

2274. MC subtype of Pleomorphic adenoma:

    I. Myxoid

    II. Cellular

    III. Classic

2275. MC malignant tumor of lacrimal gland:

    I. Adenoid cystic carcinoma (aka cylindroma)

    II. Malignant mixed tumor (aka carcinoma ex pleomorphic adenoma)

    III. Mucinous adenocarcinoma

    IV. Mucoepidermoid carcinoma

2276. MC histopathological pattern of adenoid cystic carcinoma: Cribriform with classic "Swiss cheese" appearance (Basaloid is least common)

2277. MC employed treatment for adenoid cystic carcinoma of the lacrimal gland: Combination of tumor resection with radiotherapy

2278. MC type of Ocular Adnexal Lymphoma:

    I. Primary lymphoma (78%)

    II. Secondary lymphoma (22%)

2279. MC type of Primary OAL (Ocular Adnexal Lymphomas):

MOST COMMONS IN OPHTHALMOLOGY

    I.   EMZT (Extranodal Marginal Zone Type) B cell lymphoma (41%)

    II.   Follicular lymphoma (21%)

2280. MC type of Secondary OAL (Ocular Adnexal Lymphomas): Follicular lymphoma (31%)

2281. MC location of Ocular Adnexal Lymphoma:

    I.   Orbit (64%)

    II.   Conjunctiva (28%)

    III.   Eyelid (8%)

2282. MC malignant transformation encountered in Pleomorphic Adenoma: Carcinoma ex Pleomorphic Adenoma (Malignant Mixed Tumor)

2283. MC used antilymphocyte antibody treatment for lymphoma: Rituximab (Anti CD20 antibody)

2284. MC secondary epithelial neoplasm of orbit: SCC

2285. MC orbital site of osteosarcoma: Maxillary bone

2286. MC location of Primary conjunctival cysts of the orbit: Superonasal quadrant of the orbit

2287. MC location of dermoid and epidermoid cysts of the orbit:

    I.   Superotemporal orbital rim

MOST COMMONS IN OPHTHALMOLOGY

    II.   Superonasal orbital rim

2288. MC caruncular tumors:

    I.   Papilloma

    II.   Nevus

2289. MC intrinsic tumor of the optic nerve: Astrocytoma or optic nerve glioma

2290. MC location of Eosinophilic Granuloma in orbit: Frontal bone

2291. MC location of Neurilemmoma (Schwannoma): Orbit

2292. MC structure of the eye affected in oculodermal melanocytosis: Episclera

2293. MC sinus malignancy to invade the orbit:

    I.   Squamous cell carcinoma

    II.   Inverted papilloma

2294. MC complication of Orbital Irradiation: Dry eye

2295. MC complication of orbital bone decompression surgery: Development or worsening of strabismus

2296. MC malignant tumor of parotid gland:

    I.   Mucoepidermoid carcinoma

    II.   Adenoid cystic carcinoma

2297. MC sarcoma of the orbit:

    I. Malignant fibrous histiocytoma
    II. Hemangiopericytoma
    III. Fibrosarcoma

2298. MC orbital tumor in Uganda regardless of age:
    I. Burkitt's lymphoma
    II. Granulocytic sarcoma

2299. MC cause of Hyperostosis of the orbital bones: Meningioma of the sphenoid bone

2300. MC intracranial tumor to extend into the orbit: Meningioma

2301. MC orbital bone involved by ossifying fibroma:
    I. Frontal
    II. Ethmoid
    III. Maxillary

2302. MC orbital bone involved by Intraosseous Hemangioma: Frontal bone

Uveal Melanoma

2303. MC type of uveal melanoma: Mixed cell type

2304. MC cell type in uveal melanoma: Spindle B cells

2305. MC used antigen for microvascular density of uveal melanoma: CD34

2306. MC method for treating uveal melanoma:

    I.   Brachytherapy (aka Plaque radiotherapy)

    II.   Enucleation

2307. MC used isotopes for brachytherapy of uveal melanoma:

    I.   Ruthenium-106

    II.   Iodine-125

    III.   Palladium-103

2308. MC complications of brachytherapy of uveal melanoma:

    I.   Cataract

    II.   Radiation retinopathy and maculopathy

    III.   Irradiation optic neuropathy

    IV.   Vitreous haemorrhage

    V.   Iris neovascularization

2309. MC site for metastasis in uveal melanoma:

    I.   Liver

    II.   Lung

2310. MC cause of vision loss in an eye with posterior melanoma: Retinal detachment

2311. MC indication of Transpupillary thermotherapy (TTT): As a supplement to plaque radiotherapy

2312. MC cause of secondary vision loss in stereotactic irradiation:

   I. Radiation retinopathy

   II. Opticopathy

   III. Neovascular glaucoma

2313. MC cause of secondary eye loss in stereotactic irradiation: Neovascular glaucoma

2314. MC site of metastasis of uveal melanoma:

   I. Liver (60%)

   II. Subcutaneous tissue (25%)

   III. Central nervous system (CNS) (2%)

2315. MC primary tumors associated with bilateral diffuse uveal melanocytic proliferation (DUMP):

   I. Carcinoma of the reproductive tract in women

   II. Carcinoma of the retroperitoneal area and the lungs in men

2316. MC lesions mistaken for choroidal melanoma:

   I. Choroidal nevus (27%)

   II. Congenital hypertrophy of the retinal pigment epithelium (10%)

III. Reactive hyperplasia of the RPE (6%)

IV. Rhegmatogenous retinal detachment

V. Disciform macular degeneration with extensive RPE hyperplasia (13%)

2317. MC location of Choroidal melanoma: Posterior pole

2318. MC reasons for decrease in vision in the treatment of posterior uveal melanomas:

    I. Radiation retinopathy

    II. Papillopathy

Retinoblastoma

2319. MC form of Retinoblastoma:

    I. Unilateral sporadic form (66%)

    II. Hereditary or Germ-line form (33%)

2320. MC type of somatic mutation in retinoblastoma:

    I. Point mutation

    II. Small deletions

2321. MC causes of pseudoretinoblastoma:

MOST COMMONS IN OPHTHALMOLOGY

    I.   Persistent hyperplastic primary vitreous (PHPV, Now PFV – Persistant Fetal Vasculature) (28%)

    II.   Coats disease (16%)

    III.   Presumed ocular toxocariasis (16%)

2322. MC inflammatory disease that simulates retinoblastoma: Ocular toxocariasis

2323. MC mode of presentation of retinoblastoma:

    I.   Leukocoria (56%)

    II.   Strabismus

2324. MC type of strabismus seen in retinoblastoma patient: Esotropia

2325. MC used treatment in RB patients with good prognostic factors (Reese-Ellsworth criteria Ia, Ib, IIa, and IIb): External beam radiation therapy (EBRT)

2326. MC ocular complications of external beam radiotherapy for retinoblastoma: Cataract

2327. MC secondary malignant neoplasms (SMNs) in retinoblastoma survivors:

    I.   Osteosarcoma (MC in femur bone)

    II.   Malignant melanoma

MOST COMMONS IN OPHTHALMOLOGY

2328. MC site of metastasis of retinoblastoma: Brain

2329. MC mode of extraocular extension of retinoblastoma: Periemissarial blood vessels

2330. MC cause of leukocoria in children:

    I.   Retinoblastoma

    II.   PHPV (Persistent Hyperplastic Primary Vitreous)

2331. MC primary treatment for intraocular retinoblastoma: Systemic chemotherapy

2332. MC regression pattern of retinoblastoma following primary chemotherapy:

    I.   Type III (combination of type I and type II regression)

    II.   Type I (Heavy calcification)

    III.   Type II ('fish flesh' or No calcification)

    IV.   Type IV (Flat chorioretinal scars)

2333. MC cause of type IV regression pattern in retinoblastoma: Laser consolidation

2334. MC entity confused with Toxocara canis endophthalmitis: Retinoblastoma

2335. MC inflammatory disease that simulates retinoblastoma: Ocular toxocariasis

2336. MC chemotherapy regimen for retinoblastoma: Systemic three-agent chemotherapy with carboplatin, vincristine, and etoposide

2337. MC route for retinoblastoma tumor to escape from the eye: Way of the optic nerve

2338. MC clinical classification systems used for Retinoblastoma:
   I.   Reese–Ellsworth classification (REC)
   II. International Classification (IC)

2339. MC mechanism of glaucoma in retinoblastoma: Iris neovascularization

2340. MC cause of RB protein inactivation:
   I.   Deletion
   II. Nonsense mutation

2341. MC tumor consequence to RB radiation: Osteosarcoma

2342. MC second malignancy in RB patients: Osteosarcoma of Orbit or Femur

2343. MC epithelial cancer in patients with heritable RB:
   I.   Lung cancer
   II. Bladder cancer

2344. MC source used for RB Brachytherapy: Iodine-125 and ruthenium-106

2345. MC cause of vision loss in children treated with EBRT: Retinal vasculitis

2346. MC mode of dissemination of retinoblastoma:

   I.   Through the optic nerve to brain

   II. Haematogenous spread from invasion of choroid and/or sclera, usually to bone marrow

2347. MC & dangerous route of metastasis of retinoblastoma is direct extension into the optic nerve

Rhabdomyosarcoma

2348. MC childhood orbital malignancy:

   I.   Rhabdomyosarcoma

   II. Neuroblastoma

2349. MC soft tissue tumor of childhood: Rhabdomyosarcoma (20% of all soft tissue sarcoma and 5% of all childhood cancer)

2350. MC age group affected by Rhabdomyosarcoma: 1-20 years of age

2351. MC variant of Rhabdomyosarcoma:

   I.   Embryonal (50-60% of total, mostly in children)

   II. Alveolar (aggressive with worst prognosis, mostly in adolescents)

MOST COMMONS IN OPHTHALMOLOGY

    III.   Pleomorphic or anaplastic (best prognosis, rarest, mostly in elderly)

    IV.   Botryoid (rare)

2352. MC site of origin of orbital rhabdomyosarcoma: Superior nasal quadrant of orbit (Typically it does not arise from extraocular muscles, though it may involve them)

2353. MC muscle involved in orbital rhabdomyosarcoma: Superior rectus

2354. MC site of rhabdomyosarcoma in children:

    I.   Parameninges

    II.   Orbit (though it is MC primary orbital malignancy)

Neuroblastoma

2355. MC tumor to metastasize to the orbit in children:

    I.   Neuroblastoma (40%)

    II.   Ewing's sarcoma (2nd MC)

2356. MC orbital sites of involvement of metastatic neuroblastoma:

    I.   Superolateral orbit

    II.   Zygoma with secondary extension

2357. MC primary site of neuroblastoma: Abdomen (Adrenal medulla is MC)

2358. MC sign of orbital metastatic neuroblastoma: Proptosis and periorbital ecchymosis ("panda bear eyes")

2359. MC solid tumor of the childhood: Neuroblastoma (10-15% of all paediatric cancer)

2360. MC ophthalmologic manifestations of an esthesioneuroblastoma:

   I. Periorbital pain
   II. Excessive tearing
   III. Eyelid edema

Optic Nerve Related Tumors

2361. MC intrinsic tumor of the optic nerve:

   I. Optic nerve glioma (astrocytoma) (MC in children)
   II. Optic nerve Meningiomas (MC in adults)

2362. MC Primary Tumors of the Optic Nerve Sheath: Primary optic nerve sheath meningiomas (ONSMs)

2363. MC site of optic nerve involvement in ONSM: Posterior apical aspect of the optic nerve

2364. MC optic nerve tumor of children: Juvenile pilocytic astrocytomas

2365. MC optic nerve tumor of Adult:

MOST COMMONS IN OPHTHALMOLOGY

    I.   Primary: Optic nerve Meningioma

    II.   Secondary: Leukemic infiltrates

2366. MC type of astrocytoma: Fibrillary astrocytoma

2367. MC presenting sign of Optic nerve glioma:

    I.   Proptosis (usually temporal) (94%)

    II.   Loss of vision (88%)

    III.   Optic disc pallor (59%)

    IV.   Disc edema (35%)

    V.   Strabismus (27%)

2368. MC late sign of optic nerve glioma: Optic atrophy

2369. MC symptom of optic nerve meningiomas:

    I.   gradual vision loss occurring over one to five years

    II.   Visual field loss

2370. MC growth pattern of optic nerve meningioma:

    I.   Tubular (expansion parallel to the optic nerve because of sheath confinement)

    II.   Exophytic (outpouching at the site of a break in the dura)

    III.   Fusiform (oval shape as a result of a combination of the previous two patterns)

2371. MC location of optic nerve glioma in Neurofibromatosis:

    I.   Orbital portion of optic nerve (66%)

    II.   Chiasma (62%)

2372. MC location of optic nerve glioma in patients without Neurofibromatosis: Chiasma (91%)

2373. MC secondary optic nerve malignancy:

    I.   Primary from intraocular structures (uveal melanoma and retinoblastoma)

    II.   Adenocarcinoma

Misc Eye Oncology

2374. MC extraocular association of coat's disease: Muscular dystrophy

2375. MC extracolonic manifestations of the FAP (Gardner's Disease): POFLs (Pigmented Ocular Fundus Lesions) & Opaque jaw lesions

2376. MC presenting symptom of CHR (Combined hamartoma of the retina and RPE):

    I.   Painless decrease in vision

    II.   Blurred vision

III. Floaters

2377. MC Manifestations of PCNSL-O/PIOL (Primary CNS Lymphoma with Ocular Involvement): Posterior uveitis or vitritis

2378. MC abnormality on fluorescein angiography in PCNSL-O: Punctate hyperfluorescent lesions predominantly involving the posterior pole

2379. MC malignancy affecting the vitreous: Primary intraocular lymphoma (PIOL) aka primary vitreoretinal lymphoma

2380. MC symptoms of Primary intraocular lymphoma (PIOL): Painless decrease in vision and floaters

2381. MC ocular finding of Primary intraocular lymphoma (PIOL): Hazy vitritis with clumps or sheets of vitreous cells

2382. MC ocular ultrasound finding in PIOL:

    I. Vitreous debris (77%)

    II. Choroidal scleral thickening (46%)

    III. Widening of the optic nerve (31%)

2383. MC region of brain parenchymal involvement in PCNSL: Frontal lobe

2384. MC presenting features of PCNSL: Personality alterations and changes in alertness

2385. MC type of intraocular lymphoma: Reticulum cell lymphoma

2386. MC encountered primary visual paraneoplastic disorder: Cancer-associated retinopathy (CAR)

2387. MC association of CAR (Cancer Associated Retinopathy): Small Cell Carcinoma of Lung

2388. MC auto-antibody to retina found in Cancer-associated retinopathy (CAR): Anti-recoverin antibody, which targets a 23 kD protein (recoverin) found in rods and cones

2389. MC cancer associated with Bilateral diffuse uveal melanocytic proliferation (BDUMP- rare paraneoplastic retinopathy):
   I. Male: Lung and retroperitoneal cancers
   II. Female: Cancers of the reproductive tract

2390. MC malignancy associated with Opsoclonus/saccadomania: Lung cancer

2391. MC autoantibody found in patients with opsoclonus: Anti-Ri antibody

2392. MC brain neoplasms:
   I. Gliomas
   II. Meningiomas

2393. MC treatment in patient with ocular metastasis: Radiotherapy

MOST COMMONS IN OPHTHALMOLOGY

2394. MC association with Intraocular lymphoma: Primary CNS Non-Hodgkin's B cell lymphoma

2395. MC neurologic finding in Organoid Nevus Syndrome: Seizures

2396. MC primary intraparenchymal brain tumors: Glioma

2397. MC solid neoplasms in children: Primary brain tumors

2398. MC cause of cancer-related death in children: Primary brain tumors

2399. MC type of cancer in children:
   I. Leukemia
   II. Primary brain tumors

2400. MC subtypes of leukemia affecting children:
   I. Acute lymphoblastic leukemia (ALL)
   II. Acute myelogenous leukemia (AML)

2401. MC neonatal or congenital leukemia: AML

2402. MC ocular tissue involved in leukemia clinically: Retina

2403. MC ocular tissue involved in leukemia histologically: Choroid

2404. MC ocular manifestation of leukemia: Leukemic retinopathy

2405. MC retinal findings in patients with leukemic retinopathy: Preretinal and intraretinal haemorrhages

2406. MC presenting symptom of infants with brain tumors: Vomiting

MOST COMMONS IN OPHTHALMOLOGY

2407. MC supratentorial tumors in childhood: Astrocytomas

2408. MC posterior fossa tumor in childhood: Medulloblastomas (PNETs)

2409. MC tumor of fourth ventricle:
    I.   Medulloblastoma
    II. Astrocytoma

2410. MC encountered brainstem tumor in children: Diffuse gliomas

2411. MC site of origin of brainstem gliomas:
    I.   Pons
    II. Midbrain
    III. Medulla

2412. MC tumors of pineal region: Germ cell tumors

2413. MC location of epidermoids in brain:
    I.   Cerebellopontine angle
    II. Pineal region
    III. Suprasellar area
    IV. Middle cranial fossa

2414. MC location of ganglion cell tumor: Floor of the 3rd ventricle

2415. MC sites for bone formation within the eye:
    I.   Choroid

II. Retinal pigment epithelium

2416. MC vascular tumor of the choroid: Choroidal hemangioma

2417. MC complication of circumscribed and diffuse choroidal hemangiomas: Serous detachment of the retina involving the fovea

2418. MC condition in which transvitreal biopsy is performed: Subretinal mass in the posterior pole

2419. MC malignancies to arise from radiation dermatosis:
   I. Basal cell carcinoma
   II. Squamous carcinoma
   III. Mesenchymal sarcoma

2420. MC site of origin of paraganglioma/chemodectoma:
   I. Carotid body
   II. Jugulotympanic and vagal bodies

2421. MC location of leiomyoma: Female genital tract

2422. MC location of leiomyosarcoma: Retroperitoneal

2423. MC soft tissue tumor of the body: Lipoma

2424. MC subtype of liposarcoma of orbit: Myxoid/round cell

2425. MC adult malignant soft tissue tumor in body: Malignant fibrous histiocytomas (MFH)

MOST COMMONS IN OPHTHALMOLOGY

2426. MC type of intraorbital meningioma: Intracranial meningiomas which secondarily invade the orbit

2427. MC malignant tumor among children in tropical Africa: Burkitt's lymphoma

2428. MC plasma cell dyscrasia: Multiple Myeloma

2429. MC form of eccrine carcinoma:
   I. Ductal eccrine carcinoma (generally occurs in skin of the head and neck)
   II. Eccrine porocarcinoma (generally occur on the lower extremities)

2430. MC bone affected by Infantile cortical hyperostosis (Caffey disease): Mandible

2431. MC used topical agent for atypical melanocytic lesions of conjunctiva: Mitomycin C

2432. MC tumor that may require enucleation for management:
   I. Retinoblastoma
   II. Choroidal melanoma

… MOST COMMONS IN OPHTHALMOLOGY

Optics & Refraction

General Optics

2433. MC used technique of refraction in children: Cycloplegic retinoscopy

2434. MC used cycloplegic drop in USA: Cyclopentolate

2435. MC used strength of cyclopentolate for cycloplegia: Cyclopentolate 1%

2436. MC visual acuity criteria:

   I. Detection

   II. Resolution

   III. Identification (recognition)

2437. MC measured visual function: Visual acuity

2438. MC stimuli for clinical evaluation of spatial contrast sensitivity: Repetitive patterns of alternating light and dark bars in which the luminance of the bars varies sinusoidally along a single axis

2439. MC ways by which linearly polarized light is created either in nature or in the laboratory:

   I. Transmission

   II. Reflection

   III. Scattering

MOST COMMONS IN OPHTHALMOLOGY

2440. MC difference of diopters used in defining significant anisometropia: Difference of 2 diopters

2441. MC reason why the retinoscopist may find only one meridian of a patient's astigmatism: He or she merely did not recognize the first one when it came upon

2442. MC mistake in working with vergence calculations: Ignoring the negative sign for divergent light

2443. MC instrument used in determining the astigmatic correction: Jackson cross cylinder

2444. MC sphero-cylindrical combination in cross cylinder: - 0.25 D sph with a + 0.25 D cyl

2445. MC visual impairment in humans: Presbyopia (old-sightedness)

2446. MC cause of ammetropia: Presbyopia

2447. MC defect of accommodation: Presbyopia

2448. MC undetected refractive error: Low degree of Hyperopia

2449. MC detected refractive error: Compound astigmatism (Its very controvercial as many references says its Myopia)

2450. MC cause of premature presbyopia:
   I.   Unrecognized hyperopia

MOST COMMONS IN OPHTHALMOLOGY

  II. Accommodative insufficiency

  III. Medications

  IV. Neurogenic disorders

2451. MC cause of isolated static accommodation insufficiency: Presbyopia

2452. MC therapeutic use of prisms in the orthoptics: Building up the fusional reserve of patients with convergence insufficiency

2453. MC cause of poor convergence:

  I. Senescence

  II. Lack of effort

2454. MC type of astigmatism

  I. Adults under 40 years of age: With the rule astigmatism

  II. Adults over 40 years of age: Against the rule astigmatism

2455. MC cause of astigmatism: Toricity of the anterior corneal surface

2456. MC cause of refractive headache: Uncorrected Hypermetropes

2457. MC way to correct astigmatism: Astigmatic ophthalmic lens

2458. MC astigmatic symptoms:

  I. Distortion or blurring of images at all distances

  II. Symptoms of eye strain such as headaches

  III. Photophobia

MOST COMMONS IN OPHTHALMOLOGY

    IV.   Fatigue

2459. MC objective optometer in the clinical setting: Retinoscope

2460. MC measurement of ocular refraction: Retinoscopy

2461. MC type of myopia: Youth onset myopia (aka School myopia)

2462. MC symptom of Accommodative infacility: Difficulty changing focus to various near and far distances

2463. MC used tests for determining binocular balance: Dissociation tests

2464. MC measurement of accommodation: Amplitude of accommodation

2465. MC clinical methods to quantify convergence ability: Determine the closest distance to which one can converge one's eyes (NPC: Near Point of Convergence)

2466. MC used Polarimeter or Saccharimeter: Laurent's half-shade polarimeter

2467. MC paraxial eye model used: Exact Gullstrand Eye

2468. MC used animal model for human accommodation: Rhesus monkey model

Spectacles

2469. MC method for correcting refractive errors: Spectacle lenses

2470. MC prescribed treatment for vision disorders in children: Glasses

MOST COMMONS IN OPHTHALMOLOGY

2471. MC used spectacle lens material: Normal Plastic (Previously Glass)

2472. MC used glasses for spectacle lenses: Crown

2473. MC used plastic material for spectacle lens: CR39 (Columbia Resin Type 39, RI 1.498)

2474. MC thermoplastic lens material: Polycarbonate

2475. MC used high index plastic lens material: Polycarbonate

2476. MC used high index glass lens material: Titanium glass High-Lite (index of refraction 1.701)

2477. MC plastic spectacle frame material: Cellulose acetate

2478. MC employed front curve bending for spectacle glasses: Oswalt bending (Flatter form)

(Another type of bending is Wollaston bending which is steeper form)

2479. MC method used to represent progressive addition lens designs: Contour Plots

2480. MC material used for hard coating: Lacquer

2481. MC used tint for clay shooting: Orange

2482. MC prescribed sunglass colour: Gray

2483. MC used coating material for single-layer antireflection coatings: Magnesium fluoride (MgF2, a durable substance with an index of 1.38 at 550 nm)

2484. MC coating material used for mirror coating: Chromium, aluminium, and copper

2485. MC measure of the dispersion of spectacle lenses: Abbe number

2486. MC used number for identifying the amount of chromatic aberration for a given lens material: Abbe number

2487. MC used multifocal spectacle lens: Bifocal lens

2488. MC process for adding a tint to glass lenses:

    I.   Introducing a colouring substance into the lens material before it becomes a lens

    II.   Vacuum coating the colour onto the surface of the lens in much the same way that antireflection (AR) coatings are applied to lenses

2489. MC process for adding a tint to plastic lenses: Immersion in a hot dye bath

2490. MC type of lens tint:

    I.   Solid

    II. Gradient
    III. Double gradient

2491. MC qualitative test to detect whether or not a lens is spherical: To use a lens measure in a sagittal section across the front surface (Spherical or toroidal surface will give a constant reading, whereas aspheric surface will vary in power from the centre to periphery)

2492. MC form of bifocal design: Fused bifocals

2493. MC used bifocal segments:
    I. D shaped flat top (FT)
    II. Executive
    III. C shaped curved top

2494. MC used width of Flat Top bifocals: FT28

2495. MC used trifocal design: Flat top

2496. MC task for which (Occupational Progressive Lenses) OPLs are designed and prescribed: Work at a computer

2497. MC method used to represent progressive addition lens designs: Contour Plots

2498. MC material used for hard coating: Lacquer

2499. MC method used to determine the gross axis and cylinder power: The astigmatic dial

2500. MC instrument in use for the measurement of lens power: Focimeter

2501. MC mistake made in measurement of the distance between lenses (DBL) in spectacle frame: To measure the distance between the edges of the lenses along the horizontal midline of the lens

2502. MC wrong method of measuring the effective diameter (ED) of lens shape in spectacle frame: Measuring longest diagonal of the frame shape

2503. MC method to hold lenses in eyeglass frames: To bevel the edge of the lens and place it in a frame that has a groove in the rims

2504. MC method of correcting anisometropically induced anisophoria : Reverse slab-off

2505. MC wrong method of measuring the effective diameter (ED) of a lens shape: Measuring longest diagonal of the frame shape

2506. MC mistake made in measurement of the distance between lenses (DBL): To measure the distance between the edges of the lenses along the horizontal midline of the lens

2507. MC name used for geometrical center distance (GCD):

MOST COMMONS IN OPHTHALMOLOGY

    I.   Distance between centers, or DBC

    II.   Frame PD (frame pupil distance)

2508. MC mistake in bevelling the spectacle lens: To make the bevel too pointed

2509. MC way used to hold lenses in eyeglass: Bevel the edge of the lens and place it in a frame that has a groove in the rims

2510. MC method used to make a groove into the edge of the lens:

    I.   Lens groover

    II.   Lens edger

Contact Lenses

2511. MC topographic pattern of corneal warpage: Flattening in the areas of lens bearing and relative adjacent steepening

2512. MC used surfactants in multipurpose soft lens solutions:

    I.   Poloxamine

    II.   Tyloxapol

2513. MC used soft contact lens material: Poly-HEMA (poly 2-hydroxyethyl methacrylate)

2514. MC used RGP lens material: Silicone acrylate

2515. MC type of RGP lens fit: Apical alignment fit (upper edge of the lens fits under the upper eyelid)

2516. MC type of soft contact lenses: Conventional daily reusable soft lenses

2517. MC tear reservoir depth in CONTEX lens design known as OK704T: 4D (4 dioptre)

2518. MC measure of oxygen permeability: Dk (D represents diffusion and k represents solubility)

2519. MC used contact lens design for astigmatism: Bitoric

2520. MC method of contact lens correction in presbyopia: Monovision

2521. MC used method for toric lens stabilization: Prism ballasting

2522. MC method to add a thick zone to a lens: Prism ballasting

2523. MC lens designs for correcting presbyopia:
    I.   Bifocals
    II. Progressive addition lenses (pals)

2524. MC tear proteins that deposit on soft lenses: Lysozyme and albumin

2525. MC initial base curve selected for post-LASIK contact lens fitting: 2 diopters steeper than the mean postoperative keratometric readings

2526. MC used method of determining thickness on any point of the contact: Dial gauge

2527. MC antimicrobial used in multipurpose lens solution: Polyhexanide

2528. MC used Back Optic Zone Diameter (BOZD): Between 6.0mm to 7.0mm

2529. MC pattern of epithelial keratitis seen in contact lens wearers: Fine, diffuse, superficial punctate keratitis (SPK)

2530. MC complaint with contact-lens induced nummular keratitis: Blurred vision aggravated by glare

2531. MC indication of contact lenses: Cosmetic (as an alternative of spectacles)

2532. MC uses of therapeutic contact lenses:

    I. Bandage lenses

    II. Keratoconus design lenses

    III. Rigid lenses for the correction of irregular astigmatism of various etiologies

2533. MC type of contact lens causing corneal hypoesthesia: PMMA contact lens

2534. MC method used for contact lens removal: Pinch technique

Computer Vision Syndrome

2535. MC cause of light sensitivity problems among computer users: Lighting in the work environment

2536. MC way to resolve diffuse reflection problems in computer vision syndrome: An antireflection (AR) filter placed over the computer display

2537. MC representation of the resolution of a computer monitor: Dot pitch

2538. MC distance at which people view normal hand-held reading material: 40 cm (16 in.) from the eyes

2539. MC distance of computer display: 50-70 cm

2540. MC health-related problems of computer users: Eye problems

2541. MC symptom of Computer Vision Syndrome (CVS):
   I. Eyestrain
   II. Headaches
   III. Blurred vision, dry or irritated eyes, neck and/or backaches, photophobia, double vision, and coloured afterimages

2542. MC method to reduce discomfort glare from light source: Parabolic louvers in the fixture of light

Misc Optics

2543. MC type of eye related headaches:

    I.   Frontal and brow-ache: Refractive error and convergence excess

    II.   Occipital: Convergence insufficiency and vertical imbalance

    III.   Temporal: Uncorrected oblique astigmatism

2544. MC used sans-serif letters: Sloan letters

2545. MC used clinical measure of glare: Disability glare (other types of glare are discomfort glare and light adaptation glare)

2546. MC measure used for light adaptation glare: Photostress recovery time (PSRT)

2547. MC used colour vision test: Pseudoisochromatic (PIC) plate tests

2548. MC used Pseudoisochromatic (PIC) plate tests:

    I.   Ishihara test

    II.   Hardy-Rand-Rittler test

2549. MC base direction for prism thinning: Base-down prism

2550. MC used tint in PMMA lens: Light Grey

2551. MC total corneal power: 42D (range 38D to 48D)

2552. MC value of Keratometric Index: 337.5

2553. MC used light-detection systems (or chips) in digital cameras:

    I.   CCD (charged couple device)

    II.   CMOS (complementary metal oxide semi-conductor)

    III.   Foveon

Refractive Surgery

Corneal Refractive Surgery

2554. MC refractive surgery: LASIK

2555. MC type of excimer laser: Broad beam laser

2556. MC post-operative complication with corneal lamellar flaps: Edge slippage or wrinkling of the flap.

2557. MC cause of cause of undercorrections in incisional keratotomy: Shallow corneal incisions

2558. MC employed form of incisional keratotomy: Arcuate keratotomy

2559. 2nd MC surgical procedure performed by the ophthalmic surgeon worldwide: Refractive corneal procedures

2560. MC retreatment procedure in LASIK: Re-lifting of the flap

2561. MC Deviation from optically perfect spherical (round) cornea: Regular astigmatism (with-the-rule)

2562. MC suspicious topographic findings on the anterior curvature:

  I. Corneal curvature greater than 47 D.

  II. Asymmetry between inferior and superior curvatures (I-S), where the inferior curvature is 1.4 D greater than the superior curvature

III. Skew of steepest radial axes (SRAX) greater than 20° in corneas with astigmatism greater than 1.5 D

IV. Difference in central corneal power between fellow eyes greater than 1 D.

V. Distance between the apex and the center of the cornea greater than 1 mm.

2563. MC Clinical presentation of irregular astigmatism: Spinning and scissoring of the red reflex

2564. MC used masking agent for PTK: Methylcellulose

2565. MC side effect of PTK: Hyperopia

2566. MC type of dystrophy for which PTK is used:

I. Recurrent Corneal Erosion Syndrome (RCES)

II. Granular dystrophy

2567. MC application of corneal femtosecond laser: Flap creation

2568. MC used nomogram for LRIs:

I. DONO or Donnenfeld nomogram (designed by Eric Donnenfeld)

II. NAPA or Nichamin Age and Pachymetry Adjusted nomogram (designed by Louis Nichamin)

2569. MC cause of a free cap: Flat or small cornea

2570. MC models of Intrastromal Corneal Ring Segments:

    I.   Intacs Addition Technology, Inc. (Fremont, CA, USA)

    II.   Ferrara Ring Segment (Ferrara Ophthalmics, Belo Horizonte, Brazil)

    III.   Keraring (Mediphacos, Belo Horizonte, Brazil)

2571. MC reason for a Intrastromal Corneal Ring Segment exchange: Residual myopia

2572. MC early complication after ICRS implantation: Tunnel Deposits

2573. MC late postoperative complication of ICRS: Extrusion

2574. MC centration reference used today:

    I.   Pupil centre (PC)

    II.   Corneal vertex (CV)

2575. MC formula to determine the depth of a projected ablation: Munnerlyn formula

2576. MC topographic pattern after radial keratotomy: Polygonal one

2577. MC complications of radial keratotomy: Undercorrection and overcorrection

2578. MC cause of Decentration of the Ablation:

I. Failure of the patient to fixate properly or continuously

II. Failure of the surgeon to recognize that the patient is not fixating

III. Failure of the surgeon to keep the laser centered over the entrance pupil

2579. MC used patterns for astigmatic keratotomy (AK) today:
   I. Arcuate incision
   II. T-cuts
   III. Mini Ruiz procedure

2580. MC optical zone used for ablation in myopia and myopic astigmatism: 6.0 mm

Lens Related Refractive Surgery

2581. MC surgery that corrects the refractive errors: Cataract surgery (performed five times more frequently that corneal refractive surgery)

2582. MC indications for ICL and toric ICL: High myopia and high myopic astigmatism

2583. MC complications found during implantation of ARTISAN: Iris prolapse and loss of anterior chamber depth

2584. MC used method to calculate the phakic IOL power: Van der Heijde nomogram

2585. MC wound site used for phakic IOL: Superior

2586. MC cause of elevated IOP after phakic IOL implantation: Trabecular block by viscoelastic

2587. MC complication of posterior chamber phakic IOL:
    I. Cataract formation
    II. Papillary block
    III. Glaucoma

2588. MC complaint with Phakic ACIOLs: Glare and Halos

Complications of Refractive Surgery

2589. MC patient factor associated with flap microstriae: Patients who squeezes their eye postoperatively

2590. MC early and late complication of LASIK: Dry eye

2591. MC presenting symptom of dry eye after LASIK: Visual fluctuation which is exacerbated during certain times of the day (e.g., glare at night or night vision problems)

2592. MC presentation of post-LASIK dry eyes: Corneal punctate epithelial keratopathy overlying the LASIK flap

2593. MC early postoperative complication of primary LASIK: Undercorrection

2594. MC post-operative complication after retreatment of LASIK: Overcorrection

2595. MC induced aberration after non-customised lasik: Coma

2596. MC complications of LASIK for hyperopia: Decentered ablations

2597. MC complication after surface ablation: Pain

2598. MC cause of late myopic regression: Progression of cataracts

2599. MC early postoperative complication of LASIK: Diffuse lamellar keratitis (DLK)

2600. MC Scotopic visual complaints post-refractive surgery:
   I. Nighttime starbursts
   II. Reduced contrast sensitivity
   III. Haloes

2601. MC aberration after refractive surgery:
   I. Primary spherical aberration
   II. Coma aberration

2602. MC location of epithelial ingrowth:

MOST COMMONS IN OPHTHALMOLOGY

   I.   Temporal margin of flap in nasally hinged flaps

   II. Inferior margin of flap in superior hinged flaps

   III. Rarely from center in cases of button-hole flap or central epithelial defect

2603. MC cause of DLK: Intraoperative epithelial defects

2604. MC causative organisms for infections after corneal refractive surgery:

   I.   Gram-positive cocci from the ocular adnexa (i.e. Staphylococcus aureus, Staphylococcus epidermidis, Streptococcus viridans, Streptococcus pneumoniae)

   II. Mycobacterium

2605. MC symptom of infections after corneal refractive surgery: Conjunctival injection and moderate to severe pain that persists throughout the first postoperative day

2606. MC side effect of RK: Overcorrection or undercorrections

2607. MC complication after PRK: Regression and Haze

2608. MC prophylactic treatment against excessive haze formation and regression: Corticosteroids

2609. MC cause of haze after lasik:

   I.   DLK

II. Buttonhole flaps

III. Retention of epithelial debris in the interface

2610. MC etiology of post-refractive surgery glare and haloes: Residual refractive error

2611. MC signs of infectious keratitis after LASIK: Ciliary and conjunctival hyperemia, and whitish stromal infiltrates in the interface

2612. MC finding of post-lasik dry eyes on examination: Superficial punctate keratopathy

2613. MC etiology of incomplete flaps: Microkeratome jamming (either due to electrical failure or mechanical obstacles on the microkeratome edge or footpedal)

2614. MC location of corneal infiltrates post-lasik:

   I. Flap interface
   II. Lamellar flap
   III. Stromal bed
   IV. Flap margin

2615. MC mycobacteria causing post-lasik infection: M. chelonae and M.fortuitum

2616. MC presentation of DLK at day 1: Presence of white, granular cells in the periphery of the lamellar flap, with sparing of the visual axis

2617. MC diagnosis confused with DLK: Infectious keratitis

2618. MC signs of microbial keratitis after LASIK: Ciliary and conjunctival hyperemia and whitish stromal infiltrates in the interface

2619. MC symptoms of decentered laser treatments:
   I. Blurred vision
   II. Ghosting
   III. Poor vision in low light
   IV. Glare or halo, often asymmetric around point sources of light

2620. MC clinical signs of decentration:
   I. Decreased uncorrected and BCVA
   II. Visual acuity results that vary with ambient lighting
   III. Difficult refraction or wavefront capture
   IV. Scissors reflex during retinoscopy suggestive of irregular astigmatism
   V. Significantly increased higher order aberrations of the ocular wavefront versus before surgery, especially horizontal or vertical coma

MOST COMMONS IN OPHTHALMOLOGY

VI. Abnormal corneal topography

2621. MC symptom of irregular astigmatism: Decreased in best-corrected vision and visual distortion, together with night and/or day glare

2622. MC sign of irregular astigmatism: Spinning and scissoring of the red reflex on retinoscopy

2623. MC complication following CK: Surgically induced astigmatism

2624. MC organism causing post-lasik infectious keratitis: Atypical mycobacteria and staphylococci

2625. MC source of interface debris: Meibomian gland material

2626. MC topographic abnormality seen after LASIK: Central island

2627. MC cause of central island (local steepenings of the central cornea compared with the surrounding ablated zone): Ablation for higher degree of myopia

2628. MC time of flap-displacement post-LASIK: First 24 hours

2629. MC abnormal finding on the first postoperative day of LASIK: Flap Stria (which requires flap repositioning (refloat) in up to 1% of cases)

2630. MC reported vitreoretinal complication occurring after LASIK: Retinal detachment

2631. MC complication of LASEK and Epi-LASIK: Postoperative pain

2632. MC cause of loss of BCVA after LASIK: Thin, Irregular or Buttonhole flaps

Retina & Vitreous

General Retina

2633. MC location of meridional fold: Superonasal quadrant (26% of the population, bilateral in 55%)

2634. MC location of meridional complexes: Superonasal quadrant (16% of the population, bilateral in 58%)

2635. MC form of degeneration of the peripheral retina: Typical cystoid degeneration

2636. MC location of Reticular cystoid degeneration: Inferior temporal quadrant

2637. MC location of Lattice degeneration: Superior temporal quadrant

2638. MC location of snowflake degeneration: Superotemporal quadrant (95%)

2639. MC location of tears along the anterior and posterior margins of the vitreous base:

    I. Inferotemporal

    II. Superonasal

2640. MC sign of CME in biomicroscopy: Loss of foveal depression

2641. MC Infection of Retina: Toxoplasmosis

2642. MC syndromic RP: Usher syndrome

2643. MC cause of vitreous haemorrhage:

MOST COMMONS IN OPHTHALMOLOGY

    I.   Proliferative diabetic retinopathy (32%)

    II.   Retinal tears (30%)

    III. Venous occlusions (11%)

    IV. Posterior vitreous detachments (8%)

2644. MC posterior segment finding in Systemic lupus erythematosus: Cotton-wool spots in the retina (independent of hypertension and central nervous system involvement)

2645. MC cellular components of epimacular membranes:

    I.   Fibrous astrocytes

    II.   Retinal pigment epithelial cells

    III. Fibrocytes

    IV. Myofibroblasts

    V.   Macrophages

2646. MC cause of Choroidal neovascular membranes (CNVs):

    I.   ARMD

    II.   Myopia

2647. MC cause of Choroidal neovascular membranes (CNVs) in young adults: Pathological myopia

2648. MC cause of sea-fan retinopathy: Sickle cell disease

2649. MC severe developmental anomaly in the vitreous: Persistent hyperplastic primary vitreous

2650. MC type of retinoschisis: Degenerative

2651. MC location for peripheral schisis in X linked retinoschisis:
   I.   Peripheral inferior temporal quadrant (70% of cases)
   II. Superior temporal quadrant (25%)

2652. MC type of posterior staphyloma: (total 10 types)
   I.   Disc and the macular area
   II. Macula
   III. Disc
   IV. Nasal
   V.   Inferior areas of the ocular fundus

2653. MC type of field defect in myopic eyes with posterior staphyloma: Bitemporal hemianopsia: Bitemporal hemianopsia

2654. MC encountered retinal breaks: Atrophic retinal breaks

2655. MC vision-threatening complication of high myopia: Macular choroidal neovascularisation

2656. MC retinal haemorrhage associated with hypertensive retinopathy: Superficial nerve fibre layer haemorrhage

MOST COMMONS IN OPHTHALMOLOGY

2657. MC complication when applying laser treatment for drusens in the macular area: Radial expansion of RPE atrophy from the laser lesions

2658. MC employed imaging system for Feeder vessel therapy (FVT) in CNV: High-speed dynamic video indocyanine green angiography (HSICG)

2659. MC vision-threatening macular complication in pathologic myopia (PM): Choroidal neovascularization (CNV) (4–11%)

2660. MC cause of cherry red spot in fundus:
   I. Central retinal artery occlusion (CRAO)
   II. Metabolic storage diseases

2661. MC pigmented lesion of the choroid: Choroidal nevus

2662. MC locations for retinal neovascularization:
   I. Along the vascular arcades and the optic disc (the areas of greatest adherence between the vitreous and the retina)
   II. At the border of perfused and nonperfused retina

2663. MC etiology of epiretinal membrane (ERM): Idiopathic

2664. MC indication of RETISERT (fluocinolone acetonide intravitreal implant, B & L, 0.59 mg pellet): Chronic non-infectious posterior uveitis

2665. MC etiologies of cotton-wool spots:
   I. Diabetes mellitus

MOST COMMONS IN OPHTHALMOLOGY

    II.   Systemic hypertension

2666. MC cause of metabolic vitreous opacity: Primary systemic or localized ocular amyloidosis

2667. MC cause of neoplastic vitreous opacity: Large cell lymphoma

2668. MC form of Central Serous Chorioretinopathy (CSCR):
- I. Classic or Acute CSC: Solitary, localized neurosensory detachment in the posterior pole
- II. Chronic CSC: Widespread alteration of pigmentation of the RPE in the posterior pole (aka Diffuse retinal pigment epitheliopathy DRPE)
- III. Bullous Detachment of the Retina Secondary to CSC

2669. MC angiography pattern seen with Central Serous Chorioretinopathy (CSCR):
- I. Expansile Dot Pattern (80–90%)
- II. Smokestack Pattern (10-20%)
- III. Diffuse pattern (rare)

2670. MC site of leakage in FFA in smokestack pattern of CSR: Superonasal quadrant

MOST COMMONS IN OPHTHALMOLOGY

2671. MC location of Polypoidal choroidal vasculopathy: Peripapillary and macular region

2672. MC initial symptom of Refsum Disease: Nyctalopia

2673. MC etiology for serous PED in patients less than 50 years: Central serous chorioretinopathy (CSC)

2674. MC cause of choroidal folds:
    I. Idiopathic acquired hyperopia
    II. Disciform scarring of the macula from neovascular age-related macular degeneration

2675. MC location of Idiopathic Polypoidal Choroidal Vasculopathy (IPCV) lesions: Peripapillary region

2676. MC cause of Purtscher's retinopathy: Sequela of chest-compressing trauma

2677. MC causes of retinal folds:
    I. Idiopathic epiretinal membranes
    II. Diabetic fibrovascular membranes
    III. Proliferative vitreoretinopathy

2678. MC cause of primary macular retinoschisis:
    I. Juvenile X-linked retinoschisis

II. X-linked retinoschisis (XLRS)

2679. MC cause of secondary macular schisis: Huge Myopia

2680. MC observed diseases that lead to choroidal vascular compromise:

   I. Malignant hypertension

   II. Eclampsia

   III. Severe cocaine abuse

Diabetic Retinopathy

2681. MC disorder of carbohydrate metabolism: Diabetes mellitus

2682. MC vascular complication of the diabetes: Diabetic retinopathy

2683. MC form of diabetic retinopathy: Nonproliferative diabetic retinopathy (NPDR)

2684. MC location of microaneurysms (MA) in diabetic retinopathy: Posterior pole

2685. MC cause of visual loss in patients with nonproliferative diabetic retinopathy: Macular edema

2686. MC location of Neovascularization elsewhere (NVE) in PDR: Along or just anterior to the temporal retinal vascular arcades

MOST COMMONS IN OPHTHALMOLOGY

2687. MC location of Neovascularization elsewhere (NVE) in PDR as per DRS (Diabetic Retinopathy Study):

    I.   Superotemporal quadrant (field 4, 27%)

    II.   Inferonasal quadrant (field 7, 21%)

2688. MC complications associated with visual loss in PDR:

    I.   Traction retinal detachment

    II.   Vitreous haemorrhage

2689. MC indication for vitrectomy in PDR: Diabetic tractional macular detachment

2690. MC mode of treatment for proliferative diabetic retinopathy (PDR): Laser photocoagulation

2691. MC cause of visual impairment in type I diabetics: Formation of new vessels and PDR

2692. MC cause of visual impairment in type II diabetics: Macular edema

2693. MC cause for reduction in vision following laser treatment for diabetic maculopathy: Progression in maculopathy (rather than deterioration in vision secondary to laser)

2694. MC site of extensive fibrovascular proliferations in PDR: On and near the disc

MOST COMMONS IN OPHTHALMOLOGY

2695. MC type of retinal detachment in diabetics: Nonrhegmatogenous tractional detachment

2696. MC patient group affected by diabetic Tractional retinal detachment: Young type 1 diabetic patient

2697. MC pathogenesis of bleeding in diabetic retinopathy:
   I. Retinal ischemia causing the release of angiogenic vasoactive factors
   II. Tearing of the retinal vessels caused by either a break in the retina or detachment of the posterior vitreous

2698. MC location of hard exudates in retinal layer: Outer plexiform layer

2699. MC type of cell in pancreatic islet: B (beta) cells

2700. MC used insulin regimes:
   I. An evening basal bolus (long-acting insulin) with injections of short-acting insulin before each main meal
   II. Injections of a mixture of short and intermediate insulin, the first before breakfast, the second before the evening meal

2701. MC side effect of insulin therapy: Hypoglycemia

2702. MC used insulin secretogauge drug: Sulphonylureas (SUs)

2703. MC adverse effect of Incretin mimetic group of drugs: Gastrointestinal disturbances

Age Related Macular Degeneration

2704. MC ocular condition of elderly humans with BrM (Bruch's membrane) dysfunction: Age-related macular degeneration (ARMD)

2705. MC cause of blindness in the elderly population in the western world: Age-related macular degeneration (ARMD)

2706. MC type of ARMD: Nonexudative or Dry ARMD (80-90%)

2707. MC identified clinical feature of early ARMD: Drusen

2708. MC type of drusen: Small hard drusen

2709. MC presenting symptom of choroidal neovascularization (CNV) in AMD:

    I.   Decreased visual acuity

    II.   Distortion

2710. MC cause of severe visual loss in advanced AMD: Choroidal neovascularization (CNV)

2711. MC type of neovascular lesion in ARMD: Occult form of CNV

2712. MC cellular components of CNV:

    I.   Vascular endothelium

II.   Retinal pigment epithelium

   III. Fibrocytes

2713. MC complication of Pigment Epithelial Detachment (PED): Formation of CNV

2714. MC cause of CNV: ARMD

2715. MC inflammatory condition causing CNV: Presumed Ocular Histoplasmosis Syndrome (POHS)

2716. MC manifestations of the presumed ocular histoplasmosis syndrome (POHS): Peripapillary atrophic changes and peripheral pigmented "punched-out" chorioretinal lesions without uveitis

2717. MC type of CNV in OHS: Classic CNV

2718. MC cause of RPE Tear: CNV secondary to AMD

2719. MC zinc related problem from AREDS therapy: Increased hospitalization due to genitourinary problem especially prostate enlargement

Hereditary Retinal Disorders

2720. MC hereditary hyaloideoretinopathies: Stickler syndrome

MOST COMMONS IN OPHTHALMOLOGY

2721. MC inherited cause of retinal detachment in children: Stickler syndrome

2722. MC cause of retinal detachment in Stickler syndrome: Giant retinal tears

2723. MC form of vitreoretinal degeneration: Stickler syndrome

2724. MC chondrodysplasia associated with vitreoretinal degeneration: Stickler syndrome (aka hereditary progressive arthro-ophthalmopathy)

2725. MC type of Stickler Syndrome:
    I. Type 1 - SLT I - membranous vitreous type: Mutation in the COL2A1 gene
    II. Type 2 – SLT II - beaded vitreous type: Defect in the COL11A1 gene
    III. Type 3 – SLT II - nonocular type : Defect in COL11A2 gene (systemic Stickler, without ocular)

2726. MC cause of foveal/macular hypoplasia:
    I. Albinism
    II. Rod monochromacy
    III. Aniridia

2727. MC metabolic disease causing cherry red spot: Tay-sachs disease

2728. MC flecked retinal syndrome involving the RPE: Stargardt disease/fundus flavimaculatus

2729. MC lesion mistaken for Best's disease: Yellow premacular haemorrhage

2730. MC presenting symptom of Best's disease:
   I.   Decreased visual acuity
   II. Metamorphopsia

2731. MC abnormality observed in Cone dystrophy:
   I.   Early: Pigmentary stippling with diffuse pigment granularity in the posterior pole
   II. Late: "bull's-eye" pattern of retinal pigment epithelial atrophy

2732. MC type of Pattern dystrophy:
   I.   Adult onset Foveomacular Vitelliform Dystrophy (AFVD) (MC sporadic)
   II. Butterfly shaped pigment dystrophy (BPD) (MC autosomal dominant)

2733. MC appearance of Pattern Dystrophy: Bilateral, triradiate ("butterfly") pattern of yellow or gray pigment at the level of the RPE in the central macular region

2734. MC presenting symptom of pattern dystrophies: Slightly diminished visual acuity or metamorphopsia

2735. MC form of juvenile-onset retinal degeneration in males: X-linked retinoschisis (XLRS)

2736. MC cause of spontaneous vitreous haemorrhage in young male in western countries: X linked retinoschisis (XLRS)

2737. MC complication of X-linked retinoschisis (XLRS):
   I. Retinal detachment (11%)
   II. Vitreous haemorrhage (4%)

2738. MC retinal layer involved in X-linked retinoschisis (XLRS): Outer plexiform layer (OPL)

2739. MC associated with systemic condition with Angioid streaks: Pseudoxanthoma elasticum (PXE) (Grönbald–Strandberg syndrome)

2740. MC complication of angioid streaks: Development of choroidal neovascularization (CNV)

2741. MC cause of vision loss in Birdshot chorioretinopathy (BCR): CME

2742. MC differential diagnostic consideration of Combined Hamartoma of the Retinal Pigment Epithelium and Retina (CHRRPE): Epiretinal membrane

2743. MC location of Combined Hamartoma of the Retinal Pigment Epithelium and Retina (CHRRPE): Disc margin

MOST COMMONS IN OPHTHALMOLOGY

2744. MC ocular finding associated with familial adenomatous polyposis coli (FAP): Congenital Hypertrophy of the Retinal Pigment Epithelium (CHPRE)

2745. MC presenting sign of hereditary retinal disorders: Nystagmus

2746. MC presenting symptom in North Carolina macular dystrophy: Decreased central vision

Retinal Vascular Disorders

2747. MC cause of CRAO: Carotid artery atherosclerosis

2748. MC site of occlusion in CRAO: At the level of the lamina cribrosa just before the artery enters the retina

2749. MC cause of nonarteritic CRAO and BRAO: Retinal emboli

2750. MC variant of retinal emboli:
    I.   Yellow refractile cholesterol embolus (Hollenhorst plaque) (74%)
    II. Platelet- fibrin emboli (15.5%)
    III. Calcific emboli (10.5%)

2751. MC etiology for retinal arterial occlusion:

MOST COMMONS IN OPHTHALMOLOGY

    I.   Embolism from carotid artery atherosclerosis

    II.   Arterial hypertension

    III.   Diabetes mellitus

    IV.   Valvular heart disease

2752. MC site of atherosclerosis in the neck vessels: At the origin of the internal carotid artery

2753. MC etiology for retinal arterial occlusion under age 40: Cardiac embolism

2754. MC hematologic abnormality in young patients with retinal artery occlusion: Protein S deficiency

2755. MC origin of calcific retinal emboli: Cardiac valves

2756. MC observed defect on macular visual field testing in CRAO:

    I.   Central scotoma

    II.   Paracentral scotoma

2757. MC findings in the chronic stage of eyes with CRAO:

    I.   Optic atrophy (91%)

    II.   Retinal arterial attenuation (58%)

    III.   Cilioretinal collaterals (18%)

    IV.   Macular RPE changes (11%)

MOST COMMONS IN OPHTHALMOLOGY

    V.   Cotton-wool spots (3%)

2758. MC reported visual field defects in BRAO:

    I.   Central scotoma (20%)

    II.   Inferior central altitudinal defect (13%)

2759. MC retinal vascular disease of the eye:

    I.   Diabetic Retinopathy

    II.   Branched Retinal Vein Occlusion (BRVO)

    III.   Central Retinal Vein Occlusion (CRVO)

2760. MC predisposing conditions for CRVO:

    I.   Diabetes mellitus

    II.   Arterial hypertension

    III.   Atherosclerotic cardiovascular lesions

2761. MC ocular disease associated with CRVO: Glaucoma (Glaucoma increases the risk of suffering a CRVO five to sevenfold)

2762. MC type of CRVO: Nonischemic type (75%)

2763. MC site for central retinal vein occlusion in humans: Area of the lamina cribrosa

2764. MC complication of CRVO:

    I.   Vitreous haemorrhage

II. Anterior segment neovascularization

III. Neovascular glaucoma

2765. MC complication of branched retinal vein occlusion (BRVO): Macular edema

2766. MC quadrant affected by branched retinal vein occlusion (BRVO): Superotemporal quadrant (as arteriovenous crossing sites are more frequent in the superotemporal quadrant)

2767. MC location of branched retinal vein occlusion (BRVO): Arteriovenous crossings (99% of all branch retinal vein occlusions occur at arteriovenous crossing sites with the vein posterior to the artery)

2768. MC causes of visual loss following a BRVO:

I. Macular edema

II. Macular non-perfusion

III. Vitreous haemorrhage secondary to intraocular neovascularization

2769. MC risk factors associated with BRVO:

I. Systemic hypertension

II. Diabetes

III. Hyperlipidaemia

IV. Glaucoma

V. Smoking

VI. Age-related atherosclerosis

2770. MC ocular sign of chronic carotid obstruction: Venous stasis (low-pressure) retinopathy

2771. MC hemoglobinopathy to cause retinal manifestations: Homozygous sickle cell anemia

2772. MC variant of haemoglobin in sickle retinopathy patients: Haemoglobin SC (Sickle cell anemia is severe in HbSS patients but converse is true for ocular features)

2773. MC used term for Retino-Choroidal Collaterals: Optociliary Shunt (Its actually incorrect term as there is no optic circulation, the ciliary vessels are not involved and these vessels do not take blood from an arterial to a venous circulation (a shunt))

2774. MC cause of Optociliary Shunt:

I. Central retinal vein occlusion

II. Spheno-orbital meningioma

2775. MC site of central retinal artery obstruction: At the level of the lamina cribrosa

MOST COMMONS IN OPHTHALMOLOGY

2776. MC type of parafoveal retinal telangiectasis: Idiopathic juxtafoveolar retinal telangiectasis

2777. MC form of idiopathic juxtafoveolar telangiectasis: Group 2A telangiectasis

2778. MC retinal findings in patients with leukemic retinopathy: Preretinal and intraretinal haemorrhages

2779. MC used classification for hypertensive retinopathy: Keith–Wagener–Barker classification

2780. MC retinal finding in Hypertensive Retinopathy: Retinal arteriolar narrowing

2781. MC etiology of Acute Ophthalmic Artery Obstruction: Iatrogenic sequela of retrobulbar injection (No light perception, Marked opacification with or without cherry red spot, Delayed choroidal and retinal vascular filling, decreases a and b wave on ERG)

2782. MC etiology of Combined central retinal artery and vein obstruction (CRAO and CRVA): Iatrogenic sequela of retrobulbar injection (probably by inadvertent injection into the optic nerve sheath)

2783. MC associated condition with Retinal arterial macroaneurysms (RAM): Systemic hypertension

2784. MC reported site of Acquired Retinal Macroaneurysms (RAM):

Supratemporal artery

2785. MC variants of presentation of Retinal arterial macroaneurysms (RAM):

   I.   Acute haemorrhage may develop in the subretinal space, retinal or preretinal region if the macroaneurysms ruptures.

   II. Retinal edema may be the presenting sign when chronic leakage of plasma encroaches upon the fovea.

2786. MC presentation of Retinal Macroaneurysms (RAM): Vision loss

2787. MC location of retinal haemorrhages ("salmon patches") in sickle retinopathy: Equatorial retinal periphery

2788. MC location of Sea fan fronds in proliferative sickle-cell retinopathy:

   I.   Superotemporal quadrant
   II.   Inferior temporal
   III. Superior nasal
   IV.   Inferior nasal

2789. MC location of TRD in proliferative sickle-cell retinopathy: Peripheral retina

2790. MC confused entities with the ocular ischemic syndrome (OIS):

   I.   Mild central retinal vein obstruction

II. Diabetic retinopathy

2791. MC cause of the ocular ischemic syndrome (OIS):

    I. Atherosclerosis

    II. Eisenmenger syndrome

    III. Giant cell arteritis

2792. MC sign of Ocular Ischemia: Cotton wool spots

2793. MC ocular change seen in pre-eclampsia: Focal or generalized retinal arteriolar narrowing

2794. MC manifestation of systemic hyperviscosity: Mild or "hyperpermeable," central retinal vein occlusion

2795. MC local alteration predisposing to Retinal Venous Obstruction (RVO): Open-angle glaucoma

2796. MC serious retinal vascular disease that can lead to blindness in prematurely born infants: Retinopathy of prematurity (ROP)

2797. MC zone involved with the ROP: Zone 2

2798. MC ocular complication in the CryoROP study: Intraocular haemorrhage

2799. MC type of retinal detachment in acute ROP: Tractional RD

2800. MC type of retinal detachment in chronic or cicatricial ROP: Rhegmatogenous RD

2801. MC used treatment modality for acute phase of ROP: Transpupillary laser photocoagulation delivered through indirect ophthalmoscope

2802. MC operative technique utilized for stage 4 ROP: Lens-sparing 2- or 3-port vitrectomy

2803. MC used anti–vascular endothelial growth factor (VEGF) treatment for ROP: Bevacizumab

2804.

2805. MC fluorescein angiography findings of Bechet's disease:

    I.   Diffuse vascular leakage

    II.   Hyperfluorescence of the optic disk

    III.   Hyperfluorescence of the macula

2806. MC posterior segment finding in Bechet's disease: Retinal vasculitis (intensive retinal edema, yellowish-white exudates and haemorrhages)

2807. MC ocular finding associated with Pregnancy Induced Hypertension (PIH): Focal and generalized arteriolar narrowing

Retinal Detachments
2808. MC form of retinal detachment: Rhegmatogenous RD

2809. MC cause of Rhegmatogenous Retinal Detachment (RRD): Age related PVD

2810. MC type of EDS in which Spontaneous and traumatic retinal detachment occur: EDS Type VI

2811. MC cause of failed retinal detachment surgery:
   I. MC cause of early failure: Missed breaks and redetachments
   II. MC cause of late failure: Proliferative vitreoretinopathy (PVR)

2812. MC location of Proliferative vitreoretinopathy (PVR): Inferior retinal quadrants

2813. MC inherited cause of retinal detachment in children: Stickler's syndrome

2814. MC cause of choroidal effusion/detachment: Hypotony from ocular surgery

2815. MC peripheral retinal condition that is most frequently associated with retinal detachment: Lattice degeneration

2816. MC vitreoretinal abnormality: Lattice degeneration (6-8% population)

2817. MC causes of rhegmatogenous retinal detachment in AIDS patients with viral retinitis:
   I. Acute retinal necrosis syndrome

II. Previously treated cmv retinitis

2818. MC disease confused with bullous detachment: Harada disease

2819. MC viruses capable of causing serous retinal detachment: Herpes virus family

2820. MC group of rhegmatogenous retinal detachments: Retinal detachment secondary to "U" ("horseshoe") tears

2821. MC used classification system for PVR: Retina Society Terminology Committee Classification (1983)

2822. MC primary cause of serous detachments: Choroidal vascular damage

2823. MC cause of posterior or central retinal breaks:
   I. Chronic tractional detachments
   II. Massive vitreoretinal adhesions
   III. Tractional fibrovascular proliferations

2824. MC finding in lattice degeneration:
   I. Abnormal pigmentation (82-92%)
   II. Tiny white or yellow flecks (80%)

2825. MC cause of a subsequent retinal detachment after prophylactic laser of break: Inadequate treatment anterior to the flap tear

2826. MC conditions associated with retinal detachment:

I. Myopia (40% to 55%)

II. Aphakia (23% to 40%)

III. Ocular trauma (10% to 20%)

Retinitis Pigmentosa

2827. MC mode of inheritance of RP:

    I. Sporadic

    II. Autosomal dominant

    III. Autosomal recessive

    IV. X-linked recessive (Lease common and worst prognosis)

2828. MC secondary forms of associated RP:

    I. Usher's syndrome

    II. Bardet-Biedl syndrome

    III. Senior- Loken syndrome

    IV. Abetalipoproteinemia

2829. MC cause of unilateral pigmentary retinopathy: Traumatic injury

2830. MC rod/cone dystrophy that affects the photoreceptors: Retinitis Pigmentosa (RP)

2831. MC type of cataract in patients with Retinitis Pigmentosa: Posterior subcapsular cataract (PSC)

2832. MC symptom of Retinitis Pigmentosa (RP): Nyctalopia (Night Blindness)

2833. MC abnormality of the vitreous in Retinitis Pigmentosa (RP): Presence of fine, dust-like pigmented cells released from degeneration of the RPE

2834. MC retinal dystrophy confused with Retinits Pigmentosa (RP): Cone Rod Dystrophy (CRD)

2835. MC form of unilateral pigmentary retinopathy that is referred to as unilateral RP: Diffuse unilateral subacute neuroretinitis or DUSN

Endophthalmitis

2836. MC group of organisms causing endophthalmitis: Bacteria

2837. MC organism found in Postoperative Endophthalmitis (POE)

    I. Staphylococcus species (Staphylococcus epidermidis > Staph aureus)

    II. Streptococcus species

    III. Gram-negative microorganisms (Pseudomonas aeruginosa > Proteus > Haemophilus)

    IV. Polymicroorganisms

V. Bacillus species

VI. Fungal species

2838. MC organisms found in Posttraumatic Endophthalmitis (PTE)

I. Bacillus species (Bacillus cereus)

II. Staphylococcus species

III. Streptococcus species

IV. Polymicroorganisms

V. Gram-negative microorganisms

VI. Fungal species

2839. MC cause of Bleb-associated endophthalmitis:

I. Early: Staph. epidermidis and P. acnes (Coagulase negative Gram Positives)

II. Late: Streptococcus sp. and gram-negative bacteria especially Haemophilus influenza

2840. MC cause of endogenous endophthalmitis: Fungi (Candida > Aspergillus)

2841. MC pathogen isolated in endogenous fungal endophthalmitis: Candida albicans

MOST COMMONS IN OPHTHALMOLOGY

2842. MC association in endogenous fungal endophthalmitis: Long-term intravenous line placement (>2 weeks)

2843. MC fungi causing fungal endophthalmitis:
    I.   Candida sp. (MC yeast isolates)
    II. Aspergillus fumigatus and flavus (MC mold isolates)
    III. Cryptococcus neoformans

2844. MC underlying condition associated with fungemia in patients of fungal endophthalmitis: Neutropenia

2845. MC characteristic sign of candida endophthalmitis:
    I.   Creamy white well-circumscribed chorioretinal lesions in posterior pole
    II. Yellow or white fluffy vitreous opacities

2846. MC cause of chronic/delayed onset endophthalmitis:
    I.   P. acne
    II. Fungal

2847. MC cause of endophthalmitis in children after ocular trauma: Streptococcus

2848. MC pathogens in posttraumatic endophthalmitis: Virulent Bacillus species (Bacillus cereus)

2849. MC empiric therapy for endophthalmitis: Intravitreal injection of vancomycin 1 mg/0.1 mL and ceftazidime 2.25 mg/0.1mL

2850. MC drug used in fungal endophthalmitis: Intravitreal amphotericin B

2851. MC source of endophthalmitis: Patient's periocular flora

2852. MC symptom of endophthalmitis (as per EVS):
   I.   Blurring of vision (94%)
   II. Pain (74%)

2853. MC findings in endophthalmitis:
   I.   Loss of fundus visibility (90%)
   II. Pupillary fibrin membrane (77.5%)
   III. Hypopyon (72%)

2854. MC cultured bacteria in acute-onset post-cataract surgery cases in EVS: Coagulase negative micrococci

2855. MC cause of visual loss in the EVS: Macular abnormalities

2856. MC preventive measures currently adopted for endophthalmitis:
   I.   Wide-spectrum topical antibiotics (commonly a quinolone) a few days preoperatively and cleaning with pure povidone iodine of the skin and eyelids, and diluted 50% in the

MOST COMMONS IN OPHTHALMOLOGY

conjunctival sac a few minutes before surgery to reduce counts of conjunctival flora

II. Isolating the eyelids and lashes with tape

III. Intracameral antibiotic: Cefuroxime has been found to cut the risk of endophthalmitis by fivefold but is ineffective against methicillin-resistant staphylococci, enterococci and pseudomonas. It also has to be reconstituted in a vial with the consequent risk of endophthalmitis. Moxifloxacin (Vigamox R, 0.1 ml) may also be used.

Misc Retina

2857. MC retinal condition with dark choroid: Fundus flavimaculatus

2858. MC complication associated with IOFBs: Persistent Ant/Post uveitis

2859. MC cause of Giant Retinal Tears (GRT):

   I. Idiopathic

   II. Trauma

2860. MC surgical cause of epiretinal membrane: Extracapsular cataract extraction

MOST COMMONS IN OPHTHALMOLOGY

2861. MC missed macular causes for unexplained visual loss are:

   I.   Small macular hole

   II. Subtle epiretinal membrane

   III. Diffuse macular edema

   IV. Shallow subretinal fluid

   V.   Vitreomacular traction

   VI. Occult subretinal neovascular membrane

   VII. Juxtafoveal telangiectasias

2862. MC cause of Cystoid Macular Edema (CME): Cataract surgery

2863. MC fundus abnormality in patients with orbital mass lesions: Choroidal (chorioretinal) folding

2864. MC feature of Retinal angiomatous proliferation: Presence of a serous PED with CME overlying the PED

2865. MC used lasers in photocoagulation:

   I.   Frequency-doubled Nd:YAG (532 nm)

   II. Yellow semiconductor laser (577 nm)

   III. Argon green (514 nm)

2866. MC side effects of macular laser treatment: Scotomas in laser burns close to the border of the foveal avascular zone

2867. MC form of Eales disease: Peripheral form

2868. MC presentation of Eales disease: Solid columns of sheathing in peripheral veins

2869. MC reported association of Eales disease: Systemic TB

2870. MC indication of vitrectomy in Eales disease: Persistent vitreous haemorrhage

2871. MC source of vitreous haemorrhage in Eales disease: New blood vessels formation

2872. MC signs of acute photomechanical retinal trauma: Retinal haemorrhages and/or holes

2873. MC signs of acute photothermal retinal trauma: Ophthalmoscopically visible photocoagulation burns without haemorrhage or holes

2874. MC signs of acute photochemical retinal trauma:
   I. Yellow-white small foveolar lesions in solar and welding arc maculopathy
   II. Larger often extrafoveal lesions in operating microscope and endoilluminator injuries

2875. MC location for retinal detachment to begin in ROP: Retinal ridge

2876. MC associated factors with worse visual outcomes in epiretinal membrane (ERM) surgery:
   I. Poor preoperative visual acuity
   II. Long duration of symptoms

2877. MC cause of Macular Hole Retinal Detachment (MHRD):
   I. High Myopia
   II. Blunt trauma

2878. MC lesions simulating a full-thickness macular hole:
   I. Epiretinal membranes with pseudomacular hole
   II. Impending macular holes
   III. Lamellar macular holes

2879. MC feature of radiation retinopathy: Macular edema (present in 87% of patients)

2880. MC duration in which radiation retinopathy develops after radiation: 6 months to 3 years

2881. MC reason for neovascularization in midperiphery of retina: Diabetic retinopathy

2882. MC reason for neovascularization in periphery of retina: Sickle cell retinopathy

MOST COMMONS IN OPHTHALMOLOGY

2883. MC ocular manifestation of Disseminated intravascular coagulopathy (DIC):

    I.   Bilateral serous retinal detachment

    II.   Submacular choroidal haemorrhage

2884. MC complication of Nd: YAG Laser Posterior Vitreolysis: Retinal and choroidal haemorrhage

2885. MC adverse effect of intravitreal aflibercept injection: Conjunctival haemorrhage

Sclera

Scleritis

2886. MC scleral disorder: Scleritis

2887. MC symptom for which patients with scleral disorders seek medical assistance: Pain

2888. MC type of scleral inflammation: Diffuse anterior scleritis (it is also least severe)

2889. MC associated disease with diffuse anterior scleritis: Rheumatoid arthritis (25-45%)

2890. MC associated disease with nodular scleritis: Rheumatoid arthritis (44-50%)

2891. MC associated disease with necrotizing scleritis:
    I. Wegener granulomatosis
    II. Rheumatoid arthritis
    III. Relapsing polychondritis

2892. MC disease associated with scleromalacia perforans: Rheumatoid arthritis

2893. MC systemic condition associated with scleritis: Rheumatoid arthritis

2894. MC type of scleritis seen in Rheumatoid Arthritis: Anterior scleritis

MOST COMMONS IN OPHTHALMOLOGY

2895. MC organism in postsurgical infectious scleritis: P. aeruginosa

2896. MC mode of infection in fungal scleritis: Exogenous infection via an accidental or surgical trauma

2897. MC fungi that cause scleritis: Filamentous fungi

2898. MC corneal complication of scleritis: Sclerosing keratitis

2899. MC presenting symptoms of posterior scleritis: Decreased vision and pain

2900. MC used media to store the sclera:
    I. Glycerin
    II. Ethanol

2901. MC prescribed drug for both necrotizing systemic scleritis and refractory necrotizing scleritis: Cyclophosphamide

2902. MC postoperative complication of scleral grafting: Progressive melting of the scleral graft (mostly due to inadequate immunosuppressive treatment)

2903. MC way of storage of scleral graft:
    I. Dry storage (after pretreatment)
    II. Storing the sclera graft in 90% ethanol

MOST COMMONS IN OPHTHALMOLOGY

2904. MC reason for enucleation in uncontrolled scleritis: Glaucoma with uveitis

2905. MC disease with c-ANCA (PR3-ANCA) positivity: Wegener's granulomatosis (WG) (aka Granulomatosis with Polyangitis GPA)

2906. MC disease with p-ANCA (MPO-ANCA) positivity:
  I. Microscopic polyangiitis (MPA)
  II. Focal necrotizing and crescentic glomerulonephritis

2907. MC disease with x-ANCA positivity: Chronic inflammatory bowel disease

2908. MC test used for the diagnosis of toxoplasmosis and toxocariasis: ELISA

2909. MC symptom with posterior scleritis:
  I. Decrease in vision and pain
  II. Diplopia
  III. Flashes
  IV. Tenderness

2910. MC sign with posterior scleritis:
  I. Redness related to anterior scleritis
  II. Conjunctival chemosis
  III. Proptosis
  IV. Lid swelling

MOST COMMONS IN OPHTHALMOLOGY

    V.   Lid retraction

    VI.   Limitation of ocular movements

2911. MC fundus findings in posterior scleritis:

    I.   Choroidal folds

    II.   Subretinal mass

    III.   Disk edema

    IV.   Macular edema

2912. MC cause of decreased vision in posterior scleritis:

    I.   Macular changes

    II.   Optic disc abnormalities

2913. MC infectious cause of scleritis: Herpes virus

2914. MC bacterial cause of local infectious scleritis: Pseudomonas aeruginosa

2915. MC Mycobacterium causing scleritis: M. chelonae

2916. MC fungi causing scleritis: Aspergillus

2917. MC viruses causing scleritis:

    I.   VZV

    II.   HSV-I

    III.   Mumps

MOST COMMONS IN OPHTHALMOLOGY

2918. MC type of scleritis in in patients with PAN (Poly Arteritis Nodosa): Necrotizing anterior scleritis (often associated with peripheral ulcerative keratitis (PUK))

2919. MC type of scleritis seen in zoster ophthalmicus: Nodular scleritis

2920. MC mechanism of bacterial scleritis: Scleral extension of primary corneal infections

2921. MC type of glaucoma in patients of scleritis: Closed angle glaucoma (usually occurs in patients with posterior scleritis who develop ciliary body rotation and secondary angle closure from ciliochoroidal detachment)

2922. MC type of surgically induces scleritis: Surgically-induced necrotizing sclerokeratitis (SINS)

2923. MC cause of surgically-induced necrotizing sclerokeratitis (SINS): Cataract surgery

2924. MC used graft material for surgical management of necrotising scleritis: Homologous donor sclera

Episcleritis

2925. MC cause of episcleritis: Idiopathic inflammation

2926. MC form of ocular inflammation seen in patients of SLE (Systemic lupus erythematosus): Episcleritis

2927. MC associated disease with episcleritis:

    I.   Rheumatoid arthritis (8-15%)

    II.   Herpes zoster

    III.   Rosacea

    IV.   Gout

    V.   Syphilis

    VI.   Atopy

2928. MC ocular disease associated with episcleritis: Acne rosacea

2929. MC complications seen in patients with episcleritis: Related to the use of long-term topical corticosteroids

2930. MC cause of visual loss in patients with episcleritis: Treatment-related complications

Misc Sclera

2931. MC systemic infection that may involve sclera:

    I.   Herpes zoster

    II.   Herpes simplex

III. Tuberculosis

IV. Syphilis

2932. MC ocular manifestations caused by atypical mycobacteria:

I. Keratitis

II. Scleritis

2933. MC ocular manifestation of Relapsing Polychondritis (RP):

I. Posterior Scleritis

II. Episcleritis

III. Uveitis

2934. MC acquired cause of blue sclera: Iron-deficiency anemia

Strabismus

General Strabismus

2935. MC form of strabismus: Essential infantile esotropia

2936. MC refractive error causing strabismus: Hypermetropia

2937. MC type of Pattern Strabismus (aka Alphabet Strabismus):

　　I.　V-pattern

　　II.　A-pattern

2938. MC association of V pattern strabismus: Infantile esotropia

2939. MC association of A pattern strabismus: Exotropia

2940. MC cause of Lambda pattern strabismus: Bilateral superior oblique overaction

2941. MC cause of X pattern strabismus: Large-angle exotropia

2942. MC myogenic palsy seen in ophthalmic departments: Myasthenia gravis

2943. MC type of childhood squint: Accommodative convergent squint associated with hypermetropia

2944. MC pattern of Intermittent cyclic esotropia: Alternate day deviation

2945. MC orthoptic problem:

　　I.　Convergence insufficiency

　　II.　Decompensated exophoria at near

MOST COMMONS IN OPHTHALMOLOGY

2946. MC disorder of vergence in adults:

   I. Spasm of the near reflex

   II. Divergence paresis

2947. MC cause of spasm of near reflex: Psychogenic

2948. MC ocular motor anomalies in dyslexia:

   I. Binocular instability

   II. Accommodative insufficiency

2949. MC performed tests for retinal correspondence:

   I. Afterimage test

   II. Bagolini striated glasses test

   III. Determination of the angle of anomaly on the major amblyoscope

2950. MC encountered form of acute strabismus in clinical practice:

   Strabismus after temporary occlusion of one eye in patients with no previous history of disturbance of binocular vision

2951. MC patterned strabismus:

   I. V esotropia

   II. A esotropia

   III. V exotropia

IV. A exotropia

2952. MC ocular motility defect in Grave's ophthalmopathy: Limitation of elevation

2953. MC type of cycle in Cyclic Heterotropia: 48-hour cycle

2954. MC cause of muscular asthenopia: Convergence Insufficiency

2955. MC type of error leading to inaccurate measurement of strabismus: Inadequate occlusion

2956. MC use of Diagnostic occlusion (Marlow occlusion or the Patch Test): Pre-operatively in cases of exotropia suspected to be of the pseudo-divergence excess type

2957. MC method used to determine if the diplopic patient is capable of fusion: To offset the deviation with prism in "free space" (natural viewing conditions)

2958. MC association of Anomalous correspondence in the form of acquisition of a pseudo-fovea accompanied by fusion: Esotropia ≤20Δ

2959. MC non-surgical therapy prescribed by orthoptists: Fusional vergence training

2960. MC method to build up fusional reserve: To use Prism bar

2961. MC used form of fusional reserve exercises: Free space techniques

2962. MC method to measure depth of the sensory adaptation: To introduce a neutral density filter bar between the polarized visor and the eye

2963. MC forms of sensory status in strabismus:

   I. HARC (Harmonious retinal correspondence)
   II. Global suppression
   III. Normal retinal correspondence with diplopia
   IV. Unharmonious retinal correspondence

2964. MC extraocular muscle affected in Aplasia of Extraocular Muscles: Inferior rectus

2965. MC abnormality causing Breakdown of the Binocular Alignment Control System: Absence of, or loss of, fast fusional vergence (aka fusion)

2966. MC form of Monofixation syndrome (MFS): MFS associated with small angle esotropia

2967. MC method to screen for ocular alignment: Subjective assessment of the symmetry of the corneal light reflex relative to the dark pupil

Amblyopia

2968. MC cause of decreased vision in childhood: Amblyopia (2% of population)

2969. MC preventable cause of monocular visual loss in children: Amblyopia

2970. MC form of amblyopia:
   I. Strabismic amblyopia associated with late-onset esotropia
   II. Anisometropic amblyopia

2971. MC treatment for unilateral amblyopia: Occlusion of the dominant eye with an opaque patch

2972. MC cause of visual deprivation amblyopia:
   I. Congenital or early-acquired cataract
   II. Corneal opacities

2973. MC refractive amblyopia: Hyperopic anisometropia

2974. MC use of occlusion therapy:
   I. Amblyopia
   II. Diplopia

2975. MC method by which occlusion therapy is done:
   I. Patch

II. Contact lenses (clear soft contact lens with a black pupil in the center)

2976. MC reason for ineffectiveness of patching: Non-compliance

2977. MC used form of penalization: Atropine 0.5–1% drops into the sound eye

2978. MC cause of Reverse amblyopia (Occlusion amblyopia): Full-time occlusion

Esotropia

2979. MC problem that initiates a prescription for spectacles around age 3 years: Accommodative esotropia

2980. MC form of childhood strabismus:
    I. Accommodative esotropia
    II. Intermittent Exotropia

2981. MC type of Accommodative esotropia: Refractive esotropia with high AC/A

2982. MC method used to determine whether or not the AC/A ratio is high: Clinical comparison of distance to near deviation

2983. Mc recognized risk factor for the development of accommodative esotropia: Excess hypermetropia.

2984. MC treatment for accommodative esotropia with a high AC/A: Bifocal lenses

2985. MC cause of esotropia in childhood:
   I. Accommodative esotropia
   II. Acquired nonaccommodative esotropia

2986. MC type of strabismus seen in hypothyroid patients: Esotropia

2987. MC heterotropia in patients with monofixation syndrome: Esotropia

Exotropia

2988. MC type of exodeviation that clinicians encounter:
   I. Intermittent primary exotropia
   II. Convergence insufficiency

2989. MC form of intermittent exotropia: Pseudodivergence excess exotropia

2990. MC cause of X-pattern strabismus: Patients with large-angle exotropia

2991. MC type of strabismus in children with see saw nystagmus: Exotropia

2992. MC misalignment in Crouzon's syndrome: V-pattern exotropia

2993. MC cause of constant neurogenic exotropia: Cortical visual insufficiency secondary to hypoxic-ischemic encephalopathy

2994. MC surgical procedure for pseudodivergence excess exotropia:

Symmetric recession of both lateral rectus muscles

2995. MC cause of Sensory Exotropia: Anisometropic amblyopia

2996. MC cause of consecutive exotropia: Prior surgery for esotropia

Fourth Nerve Palsy

2997. MC cause of 4th nerve palsy in adults:

    I.   Trauma (unilateral or bilateral fourth nerve palsy)

    II.   Decompensation of a congenital fourth nerve palsy

2998. MC cause of 4th nerve palsy in children:

    I.   Congenital

    II.   Idiopathic

    III.   Acquired

2999. MC cause of acquired 4th nerve (trochlear) palsy: Head Trauma

3000. MC single cause of a head tilt: Superior oblique palsy (SOP)

3001. MC presenting sign of Congenital Superior Oblique Paresis: Head tilt opposite to the side of the palsy

3002. MC non-traumatic mechanism 4th nerve (trochlear) palsy: Congenital anomaly of the superior oblique muscle or its tendon

3003. MC isolated cranial nerve palsy: 4th nerve (trochlear) palsy

3004. MC cause of vertical strabismus encountered in the clinical practice: Superior oblique palsy (SOP)/ 4th nerve (trochlear) palsy

3005. MC isolated cranial palsy of an extraocular muscle that requires surgery: Superior oblique palsy (SOP)

3006. MC cranial nerve paralysis encountered in ophthalmology: Superior oblique palsy (SOP)

3007. MC cyclovertical muscle palsy: Superior oblique palsy (SOP)

3008. MC used primary surgical procedure for Superior oblique palsy (SOP): IO weakening operations

Sixth Nerve Palsy

3009. MC acquired palsy: Six nerve palsy

3010. MC associated feature of Möbius syndrome (Congenital facial diplegia): Abducens palsy

3011. MC ocular motor nerve paresis that occurs in patients with a direct carotid-cavernous fistula: Abducens nerve paresis

3012. MC presentation of Moebius Syndrome: Bilateral sixth cranial nerve palsy

3013. MC cause of sixth nerve palsy in children:

MOST COMMONS IN OPHTHALMOLOGY

    I.   Trauma

    II.   Post-viral

    III.   Neoplasm

3014. MC neoplasm causing sixth nerve palsy in children: Brainstem glioma

3015. MC cause of 6th nerve deficit in individuals over age 50 years: Vasculopathic cranial neuropathy

3016. MC cause of 6th nerve palsy in children: Tumors

3017. MC intracranial mass producing 6th nerve palsy in children: Pontine glioma

3018. MC congenital ocular palsy: 6th nerve palsy

3019. MC application of Botox-A in cranial nerve palsy: Acute phase of sixth nerve palsy

3020. MC surgical approach for total sixth nerve palsy: Total vertical rectus muscle transposition to the lateral rectus insertion

3021. MC strabismus indication for use of botulinum: Sixth nerve palsy

Third Nerve Palsy

3022. MC causes of paediatric third nerve palsy:

    I.   Idiopathic congenital onset

MOST COMMONS IN OPHTHALMOLOGY

II. Head trauma

3023. MC cause of acquired oculomotor palsy: Injury (generally intracranial)

3024. MC identifiable cause of acquired 3rd nerve palsy in adults: Vascular insufficiency due to diabetes, hypertension, or atherosclerosis

3025. MC identifiable cause of acquired 3rd nerve palsy in children: Trauma

3026. MC site of lesion in an isolated acquired oculomotor paresis: In the subarachnoid space

3027. MC cause of subarachnoid oculomotor palsy: Posterior communicating artery (PCA) aneurysm

3028. MC mechanism of oculomotor paresis: Microvascular ischemia of the oculomotor nerve arising from small-vessel disease of the vasa vasorum supplying the third nerve

Duane Retraction Syndrome

3029. MC congenital cranial dysinnervation disorder (CCDD): Duane's Retraction syndrome (DRS)

3030. MC paediatric disorder associated with an isolated abduction deficit: Duane's Retraction syndrome (DRS)

3031. MC used classification for Duane's Retraction syndrome: Huber's classification

3032. MC type of Duane's Retraction syndrome: (based on electromyography)

   I. Type I (78%): Limited abduction but normal or only slightly limited adduction

   II. Types III (15%): Limited adduction but normal or only slightly limited abduction

   III. Type II (7%): Adduction and abduction are both limited

3033. MC eye involved in Duane's Retraction syndrome (DRS): Left eye

3034. MC type of strabismus seen in DRS:

   I. Esotropia (MC with type I DRS)

   II. Orthotropia

   III. Exotropia (MC with type II DRS)

3035. MC type of refractive error associated with DRS:

   I. Hypermetropia or hypermetropic astigmatism (31.5%)

   II. Myopia or myopic astigmatism (22%)

3036. MC indication for surgical treatment in Duane's Retraction syndrome (DRS): An unacceptable face turn secondary manifestation of strabismus in primary position

3037. MC adverse outcome after surgical treatment of Duane's syndrome: Undercorrection of primary position esotropia and the face turn

3038. MC recommended surgery for type 2 Duane retraction syndrome: Recession of the lateral rectus muscle on the involved side in proportion to the size of the exotropia (resection of the medial rectus muscle is avoided)

Dissociated Deviation

3039. MC hyperdeviation seen in a strabismus practice: Dissociated Vertical Deviation (DVD)

3040. MC presentation for DVD: For one eye to have a hypertropia that is intermittently manifest and for the other to have a hypertropia that is latent

3041. MC association of Dissociated Vertical Deviation (DVD): Infantile esotropia

3042. MC procedures currently used for the surgical treatment of DVD:
   I. Bilateral superior rectus recession
   II. Bilateral inferior oblique recession/anterior transposition

3043. MC indication for the inferior oblique anterior transposition procedure: DVD with significant inferior oblique overaction in the same eye

3044. MC technique used to treat Dissociated Horizontal Deviation (DHD): Graded unilateral lateral rectus (LR) recession (Bilateral LR recession is indicated when XT is bilateral; unilateral or bilateral MR recession when the patient exhibits ET instead of XT)

Misc Strabismus

3045. MC ocular causes of abnormal head posturing:
   I. Nystagmus with a null point
   II. Incomitant strabismus with compensatory head posturing to allow fusion

3046. MC type of restrictive component in paralytic strabismus: Contracture of the antagonist muscle

3047. MC compensatory head posture in nystagmus: Face turn (Right/Left)

3048. MC used subjective dissociated phoria in optometric practice: Von Graefe test

3049. MC example of pseudostrabismus: Diagnosis of pseudoesotropia in infants with large epicanthal folds

3050. MC cause of ocular upshoot in adduction: Inferior oblique overaction

3051. MC indications for surgery on the inferior oblique muscle:

MOST COMMONS IN OPHTHALMOLOGY

    I.   Superior oblique palsy

    II.   Primary inferior oblique overaction

    III.   V-pattern horizontal strabismus with inferior oblique overaction

    IV.   Dissociated vertical deviation associated with inferior oblique overaction

3052. MC way to perform Inferior oblique weakening procedure: Recession or myectomy

3053. MC indication of Full Tendon Transposition procedure: LR paralysis

3054. MC type of CFEOM:

    I.   Type 1 (Autosomal dominant type, presents with bilateral ptosis, eyes fixed in a depressed position, and variable horizontal duction deficits)

    II.   Type 2 (Autosomal recessive type, bilateral ptosis and a large-angle exotropia, with associated vertical duction deficits)

    III.   Type 3 (Autosomal dominant type, variable presentation)

3055. MC involved muscle in CFEOM:

    I.   Levator

    II.   Inferior rectus

    III.   Lateral Rectus

3056. MC developmental cause of CFEOM: Abnormality in the development of the extraocular muscle lower motor neurons, with agenesis of the third nerve being most common

3057. MC cause of Central Disruption of Fusion (Horror Fusionis): Severe closed head injury

3058. MC cause of Skew deviation:
   I.   Brain stem Infarctions and haemorrhages
   II. Tumors and multiple sclerosis

3059. MC cause of convergence spasm: Psychogenic

3060. MC cause of acquired central disruption of fusion: Moderate to severe closed head trauma

3061. MC cause of constant neurogenic exotropia: Cortical visual insufficiency secondary to hypoxic-ischemic encephalopathy

3062. MC accompaniment of strabismus: Latent nystagmus

3063. MC congenital anomalies of the extraocular muscles:
   I.   Agenesis
   II. Anomalous insertions or origins
   III. Adherence and fibrosis syndromes

3064. MC ocular manifestation of a mucocele of the maxillary sinus: Upward displacement of the eye

3065. MC measurements of saccadic dynamics: Peak velocity and duration

3066. MC cause of Dysmetria (Abnormal saccadic amplitude): Cerebellar disease

3067. MC abnormality on Maddox Rod testing in Superior oblique palsy: Excyclotorsion of the paretic eye

3068. MC motility problem in cranial dysostosis: V-pattern strabismus with severe oblique muscle dysfunction

3069. MC craniosynostosis syndrome:
   I. Crouzon's Syndrome (aka hereditarily craniofacial dysostosis with birth prevalence of 16.5 per million and 4.8% of all cases of craniosynostosis)
   II. Apert's syndrome

3070. MC type of craniosynostosis: Scaphocephaly (Sagital suture synostosed)

3071. MC misalignment in Crouzon's syndrome: V-pattern exotropia

3072. MC cervical anomaly in Crouzon's syndrome: C2-C3 fusion

3073. MC ophthalmic features of Crouzon syndrome: Hypertelorism and proptosis with inferior scleral show (lower eyelid below limbus)

3074. MC cause of teleorbitism: Craniofacial synostosis

3075. MC cause of Brown Syndrome: Congenitally tight superior oblique muscle tendon complex (termed true congenital Brown syndrome)

3076. MC cause of torticollis:
   I. Ocular torticollis
   II. Skeletal torticollis

3077. MC cause of Head Tilt in children: Congenital fourth nerve palsy

3078. MC cause of Face Turn in children: Duane syndrome

3079. MC muscle affected by Pulled-in-two syndrome (PITS) (Dehiscence of a muscle during surgery): Inferior rectus

Surgery

General Eye Surgery

3080. MC ophthalmic surgery:

    I.   Cataract surgery

    II.   Laser vision correction

    III. Vitreoretinal surgery

3081. MC used concentration of povidone-iodine for antisepsis: 5%

3082. MC positioning error the beginning surgeon makes when operating from the temporal position: Failing to raise the bed high enough

3083. MC cause of poor hand position: Lifting the hands

3084. MC cause of excessive side-to-side eye movement: Failure to keep the surgical instrument centered in the incision

3085. MC type of needle used in ophthalmology: 3/8 needle

3086. MC antiseptic agents used in preoperative preparation of the surgical site:

    I.   Iodophors (Povidone-iodine)

    II.   Alcohols

    III. Chlorhexidine gluconate

MOST COMMONS IN OPHTHALMOLOGY

3087. MC surgery causing Oculocardiac Reflex (OCR): Strabismus surgery

3088. MC cardiac response to oculocardiac reflex (OCR):
   I. Bradycardia (at least 20% decrease in heart rate from baseline)
   II. Dysrhythmias
   III. Sinoatrial arrest

3089. MC used topical ophthalmic anesthetic agents: Proparacaine 0.5% and tetracaine 0.5%

3090. MC used regional ophthalmic anesthetic agents:
   I. Lidocaine (Xylocaine) 2% to 4%
   II. Bupivacaine (Marcaine) 0.75%
   III. Mepivacaine (Carbocaine) 2%
   IV. Etidocaine (Duranest) 1.5%

3091. MC way to mechanically control intraocular bleeding: Raising intraocular pressure by mechanical tamponade

3092. MC error in any type of suture placement: Tying a suture too tight

3093. MC suture material used for iris suture: Polypropylene

3094. MC form of wound closure: Single interrupted suture

3095. MC intraocular surgery predisposing suprachoroidal surgery: Glaucoma filtering surgery (previously cataract surgery)

3096. MC used quadrant for sub tenon's anaesthesia: Inferonasal

Conjunctival Surgery

3097. MC performed technique for a total conjunctival flap: Gunderson's Flap

3098. MC intraoperative complication of conjunctival flap surgery: Formation of a buttonhole in the Conjunctival flap

3099. MC postoperative complication of conjunctival flap surgery: Retraction of flap

3100. MC indications for a conjunctival flap: Persistent, noninfected corneal ulcerations that do not respond to lubrication, patching, bandage contact lens, moist chamber, or temporary tarsorrhaphy

3101. MC indication for the use of a conjunctival flap in the treatment of infectious diseases: Herpetic keratitis (Metaherpetic and stromal keratitis)

3102. MC corneal disease associated with pain in which a conjunctival flap can be useful: Bullous keratopathy due to Fuchs' dystrophy or related to cataract surgery

Lens, IOL & Cataract Surgery

3103. MC surgical procedure in ophthalmology in patients over 60 years of age: Cataract surgery

3104. MC surgical procedure in the aged population: Cataract Surgery

3105. MC indication of cataract surgery: Visual rehabilitation/ patient's desire for improved vision

3106. MC incision used in modern phacoemulsification: Clear corneal incision

3107. MC postoperative complication with secondary IOLs:
   I.   Persistent cystoid macular edema
   II. Glaucoma

3108. MC time of PC tear while phacoemulsification: While cortical clean-up (when the flaccid capsule can easily become incarcerated in the aspiration port and torn by minor traction)

3109. MC IOL used in secondary implantation is the three-piece AcrySof IOL

3110. MC complication of SFIOLs: Polypropylene suture erosion

3111. MC timing of suprachoroidal haemorrhage in cataract surgery: After the nucleus has been removed, just before implantation of the IOL, when the eye is at its softest and has been manipulated during the preceding surgery

3112. MC method used in clinic for toric IOL alignment: Slit-lamp with rotating slit

3113. MC cause of Toric IOL rotation following an uncomplicated cataract surgery: Capsular bag shrinkage due to fibrosis

3114. MC cause of unexpected vision loss following cataract surgery: CME

3115. MC preexisting condition to result in disappointing postoperative vision following cataract surgery: ARMD

3116. MC used capsulorrhexis forceps: Kraff-Utrata capsulorrhexis forceps

3117. MC applied capsulorrhexis technique: The forceps technique

3118. MC capsulorrhexis complication: Radial tear

3119. MC reference used while performing capsulorrhexis: Pupil margin

3120. MC modification used for manual CCC (continuous curvilinear capsulorhexis): TIPP technique (two-incision push-pull technique, An MVR blade or a cystotome is used to puncture the anterior capsule at the superior and inferior ends of the planned CCC. The superior flap is pushed down and the inferior flap is pulled up until they meet each other.)

3121. MC problems identified after capsulorrhexis:

MOST COMMONS IN OPHTHALMOLOGY

    I.   Anterior capsule contraction

    II.   Incarceration of viscoelastic

3122. MC capsule staining dye used today: Trypan blue

3123. MC error made to crack nucleus after trench: Failure to place both of the instruments at the base of the groove

3124. MC cause of cracking difficulties with hard nuclei: Insufficient depth of the grooves

3125. MC used IOL material: Foldable Hydrophobic Acrylic

3126. MC positive dysphotopsia after cataract surgery: Edge glare

3127. MC used model of CTS (Capsular Tension Segment): Model 6D (4.75mm)

3128. MC performed procedure by cataract surgeon to reduce astigmatism: Peripheral arcuate corneal incisions placed on the steep axis (limbal relaxing incisions (LRIs))

3129. MC mistake novice LRI surgeons make: Not to press the LRI blade firmly against the cornea, which results in a shallow ineffective incision

3130. MC sign of good hydrodelineation: Circumferential golden ring

3131. MC reason for a complication to occur during cataract surgery: Poor visibility

3132. MC reason of PCR while IOL implantation: Not fully inflating the AC and bag with OVD prior to IOL implantation

3133. MC cause of PCR while nucleus emulsification: Post Occlusion Surge (POS)

3134. MC step in which PCR occur during phacoemulsification:
   I. Learning surgeon: Nuclear emulsification
   II. Experienced surgeon: Irrigation & Aspiration

3135. MC sign of PCR:
   I. Deepening of the anterior chamber and shift of the iris-lens diaphragm backwards
   II. Loss of followability

3136. MC causes of patient dissatisfaction after cataract surgery:
   I. Residual refractive error
   II. Ocular surface problems
   III. Posterior capsular opacification (PCO)
   IV. IOL decentration
   V. Cystoid macular edema (CME)
   VI. Dysphotopsia
   VII. Night vision problems

VIII. Problems with adaptation to the optics

3137. MC complication of cataract surgery with IOL implantation: PCO

3138. MC reason for IOL explantation:

    I. Incorrect IOL power

    II. Dislocation/decentration of IOL

    III. IOL calcification

    IV. Glare/optical aberrations

3139. MC reason for exchanging Multifocal IOLs:

    I. Unwanted visual images or dysphotopsia, such as intolerable glare and halos

    II. Poor quality of vision

3140. MC associated conditions with late spontaneous dislocation of the entire lens-bag complex:

    I. PXF

    II. Vitreoretinal surgery

3141. MC management of dislocated bag-IOL complex: Removal of the complete bag-IOL complex and implantation of a new IOL

3142. MC reason for IOL decentration: One haptic in bag and one in sulcus (IOL decenters towards the haptic in sulcus)

3143. MC reason for IOL dislocation: Inadequate capsular support

3144. MC cause of intracapsular IOL dislocation: Zonular degradation associated with pseudoexfoliation syndrome

3145. MC cause of extracapsular IOL dislocation: Sulcus placement of an inadequately sized IOL

3146. MC presenting signs and symptoms of IOL dislocation: Glare, halos, edge effect, reduced visual acuity, monocular diplopia

3147. MC symptom of IOL decentration: Unwanted optical images caused by the edge of the IOL optic

3148. MC indication of anterior vitrectomy:
    I. capsular rupture during cataract surgery
    II. surgery for anterior segment trauma

3149. MC damaged part with the vitreous cutter in anterior vitrectomy: Anterior capsule

3150. MC incisions made to perform cataract surgery with phacoemulsification: Sutureless clear corneal

3151. MC type of fluid pump used in phaco machines: Peristaltic

3152. MC indication of standard CTR (Capsular Tension Ring):
    I. Pseudoexfoliation syndrome

MOST COMMONS IN OPHTHALMOLOGY

    II.   High myopia

    III.   Subluxated lens including traumatic cataract with zonular dialysis

    IV.   Marfan's syndrome

3153. MC injector used for CTR insertion: Geuder CTR injector

3154. MC used size of CTR: 12/10 mm and 13/11 mm

3155. MC intraoperative complication of cataract surgery: Rupture of the posterior capsule with or without vitreous prolapse

3156. MC employed combined cataract and glaucoma surgery: Phacoemulsification technique combined with trabeculectomy

3157. MC method used to determine IOL power: SRK formula

3158. MC IOLs in which glistening is seen: Hydrophobic acrylic

3159. MC used intracameral anaesthesia in cataract surgery: Preservative free lidocaine 1% 0.1 to 0.5 mL

3160. MC method used to manufacture silicone IOLs: Injection molding

3161. MC silicone in silicone IOLs: Elastomers baged on the dimethylsiloxane backbone

3162. MC used irrigation solution in cataract surgery:

    I.   Past: Lactated ringer

II. Present: BSS and BSS Plus

3163. MC type of IOL resulting with dissatisfied patients: Multifocal IOLs

3164. MC used mechanical strategy for pupil expansion during IFIS: Iris retractors

3165. MC used strategies to manage IFIS:
    I. Healon 5 (60%)
    II. Iris retractors (31%)
    III. Preoperative atropine (5%)
    IV. Pupil expansion rings (4%)

3166. MC complication of IFIS cataract surgery: Mild or moderate iris defect

3167. MC cause of positive pressure in cataract surgery: Pressure on the lids and drape from the lid speculum

3168. MC used method to correct Post-cataract Surgery Refractive Surprise: IOL exchange

3169. MC cause of iris prolapse while phacoemulsification: Poorly constructed wound architecture

3170. MC causes of capsular tears during hydrosteps:
    I. Noncontinuous capsulorrhexis—visible or occult
    II. Pseudoexfoliation with friable capsule and weak zonules

III. Mature cataract with poor view of the anterior capsule

IV. Relatively small rhexis in relation to maturity of the cataract

V. Overzealous hydrodissection

VI. Viscodissection

VII. Calcified posterior polar cataracts

3171. MC cause of difficulty in removing first quadrant in phaco:

I. Interlocked posterior plate edges

II. Short troughs with interlocked peripheral edges

III. Incomplete splitting of the posterior plate itself

3172. MC cause of Descemet's membrane detachment (DMD): Dull blade

3173. MC cause of problem during foldable IOL implantation:

I. Poor loading of the implant

II. Attempt to place the lens through too small an incision

3174. MC type of phaco tip used: 30 degree tip

3175. MC causes of lens quake inducement failure: Releasing the vacuum after the tip is placed into position and occluded

3176. MC complication in the small incision cataract extraction by manual phacocracking: Corneal edema

3177. MC used dispersive viscoelastic agent: HPMC

3178. MC ocular toxic effect of viscoelastic agents: Elevated IOP

3179. MC complication during wound construction in cataract surgery: Premature entry into the anterior chamber

3180. MC type of IOLs in which Anterior Capsular Contraction Syndrome (ACCS) is seen: Silicone plate haptic lenses

3181. MC postoperative complication reported after implantation of the full sized black aniridia IOL: Elevated IOP

3182. MC postoperative complication demanding treatment following phacoemulsification: Elevated IOP

3183. MC time period when elevated IOP occur post phacoemulsification: 8-12 hours after surgery

3184. MC indication of Glued IOL:
   I. Posterior capsular rupture with no sulcus support (56%)
   II. Subluxated cataract (21%)

3185. MC cause of shallow AC with low IOP after cataract surgery: Wound leak

3186. MC cause of corneal endothelial decompensation after cataract surgery: Surgical trauma

3187. MC used aspiration tip size in IA handpiece: 0.3 mm

3188. MC complication of piggy-back implantation of IOL: Interlenticular opacification which may cause hyperopic shift and decrease in vision and IOL anterior displacement

3189. MC cause of thermal injury in phacoemulsification:
   I.   Reduced irrigant inflow
   II. Obstructed outflow

3190. MC cause of outflow obstruction causing thermal injury in phaco: Visco-obstruction

3191. MC serious intraoperative complication of cataract surgery: Posterior capsule rupture

3192. MC cause of severe eye pain within 24 hours after phacoemulsification:
   I.   Corneal abrasion
   II.   Elevated iop
   III. Suprachoroidal effusion
   IV.   Haemorrhage from hypotony

3193. MC cause of angle-closure glaucoma following cataract surgery with or without IOL implantation: Pupillary block

3194. MC complication of sulcus-sutured PC IOLs: Suture erosion

3195. MC problem faced by learning phaco surgeons: Reluctance to sculpt deeply enough

3196. MC intraoperative complication of phacoemulsification and extracapsular cataract surgery: Vitreous loss

3197. MC mechanism of vitreous loss during phacoemulsification:
   I. Extension of an anterior capsular tear through the zonule into the posterior capsule
   II. Direct injury of the posterior capsule by the tip of the phaco needle

3198. MC mistake in main incision during phacoemulsification: Going more limbal which leads to iris prolapse

3199. MC cause of Iris chaffing during phacoemulsification: Semidilated pupil and iris captured by phaco probe

3200. MC problem encountered by most of the surgeons during cataract extraction surgery: Small pupil

3201. MC surgery causing Brown-McLean syndrome (peripheral corneal edema with a clear central cornea): Intracapsular cataract surgery

3202. MC cause of UGH (uveitis-glaucoma-hyphema) syndrome: Sulcus placement of a single-piece acrylic IOL

Glaucoma Surgery

3203. MC used antiproliferative agents in glaucoma surgery:

   I.   Mitomycin C (MMC)

   II. 5-Flurouracil

3204. MC method of MMC administration in glaucoma surgery: Placing a surgical sponge soaked in MMC within the subconjunctival space in contact with sclera at the planned trabeculectomy site

3205. MC side effects of postoperative subconjunctival 5-FU injection:

   I.   Corneal and conjunctival epithelial toxicity

   II. Corneal epithelial defects

   III. Abrasion

   IV. Primary conjunctival wound leaks

3206. MC used concentration of 5-FU: 50 mg/ml

3207. MC used concentration of mitomycin C in glaucoma surgery: 0.4 mg/ml

3208. MC use of vertical mattress suture in ophthalmology: Closing a lacerated (or incised) eyelid margin, where it provides strength as well as an everting tendency, preventing an eyelid margin "notch"

3209. MC complication of deep sclerectomy surgery:

MOST COMMONS IN OPHTHALMOLOGY

    I.   Inability to find Schlemm's canal

    II.   Perforation of the sclerodescemetic membrane

3210. MC complications reported with the Trabectome:

    I.   Transient postoperative hyphema

    II.   Peripheral anterior or goniosynechiae

    III.   Transient corneal injury

    IV.   Descemet's detachment and haemorrhage

    V.   Persistent Descemet's injury

    VI.   Inadvertent iris injury

    VII.   Transient early hypotony

3211. MC procedure performed for chronic forms of glaucoma:

Trabeculectomy

3212. MC cause of failure of filtering glaucoma surgery: Subconjunctival scarring

3213. MC postoperative complication of iStent surgery:

    I.   Malpositioning of stent

    II.   Stent lumen obstruction

3214. MC early complications in trabeculectomy:

    I.   Hyphema (24.6%)

II. Shallow anterior chamber (23.9%)

III. Hypotony (24.3%)

IV. Wound leak (17.8%)

V. Choroidal detachment (14.1%)

3215. MC late complications of trabeculectomy:

I. Cataract (20.2%)

II. Visual loss (18.8%)

III. Iris incarceration (5.1%)

IV. Encapsulated bleb (3.4%)

3216. MC cause of vision loss after trabeculectomy: Cataract development

3217. MC cause of hypotony with flat AC after glaucoma surgery:

I. Over-filtration

II. Bleb leak

3218. MC mechanism of wound and bleb leak: Inadequate conjunctival closure

3219. MC complications affecting all patients after cyclophotocoagulation:

I. Mild pain lasting less than 1 day

II. Mild uveitis

III. Transient conjunctival burns and edema

3220. MC intraoperative complication of viscocanalostomy or deep sclerectomy: Perforation of Trabeculo-Descemet's membrane (TDM)

3221. MC cause of failure to identify Schlemm's canal during viscocanalostomy or deep sclerectomy: Inadequate deep dissection

3222. MC early postoperative complication of canaloplasty: Hyphema/ Hematic Tyndall

3223. MC cause of hyphema after canaloplasty: Episcleral reflux from hypotony

3224. MC postoperative complication of deep sclerectomy: Hyphema

3225. MC complication after laser suture lysis in filtration glaucoma surgery: Over filtration causing hypotony

3226. MC complication of gonioscopic stent surgery: Loss of trabecular area viewing due to bleeding caused by a failed attempt at stent insertion

3227. MC forceps used for peeling of the inner wall of SC (Schelmm's canal): Mermoud forceps

3228. MC used implant as space-maintaining device in NPGS (Nonpenetrating Glaucoma Surgeries) : AquaFlow Collagen Drainage Device

3229. MC used NPGS techniques:

    I. Deep sclerectomy

MOST COMMONS IN OPHTHALMOLOGY

    II.   Viscocanalostomy

3230. MC used glaucoma surgery:

    I.   Trabeculectomy

    II.   Glaucoma drainage device implantation

3231. MC adverse events with iStent surgery:

    I.   Elevated IOP (4.3%)

    II.   Stent obstruction (4.3%)

    III.   Stent malposition (2.6%)

3232. MC cause of increased IOP during the first week after filtration glaucoma surgery: Scleral flap that is too tightly sutured

3233. MC used animals to model glaucoma filtration surgery and ocular wound healing:

    I.   Monkeys

    II.   Rabbits

3234. MC location of buttonhole leaks in glaucoma filtration surgeries: At limbus

3235. MC step in filtration glaucoma surgery when intraoperative anterior chamber haemorrhage can occur: At the time of iridectomy

3236. MC appearance of decompression retinopathy seen after glaucoma surgery: Appearance like CRVO

3237. MC late postoperative complication of glaucoma surgery: Filtration failure due to fibrosis

3238. MC mechanism of early filtration failure: Occlusion at internal sclerostomy site

3239. MC mechanism of late filtration failure in glaucoma surgery: Scarring at the Conjunctiva-Tenon's capsule-Episcleral interface

3240. MC used manoeuvre to improve the surgical success in the postoperative management of trabeculectomies: Ocular massage

3241. MC described sign reported to influence bleb failure: Bleb vascularity

3242. MC sign associated with a good outcome of bleb: Presence of microcysts

3243. MC complication of laser filtration procedures (Ab interno Nd: YAG laser sclerostomy): Iris incarceration

3244. MC complications of cyclocryocoagulation:
    I. Intense postoperative pain for several days
    II. Transient iop elevation
    III. Hyphaema

IV. Secondary uveitis

3245. MC used nonvalved tube shunts:

    I. Molteno (Molteno Ophthalmic Ltd, Dunedin, New Zealand)

    II. Baerveldt (Abbott Medical Optics, Santa Ana, CA)

3246. MC used valved tube shunts: Ahmed design (New World Medical, Inc, Rancho Cucamonga, CA)

3247. MC device related complication of Ex-PRESS glaucoma shunt: Blockage of the lumen of the implant (can effectively be treated with Nd:YAG laser treatment of the tube tip in the anterior chamber)

3248. MC shunt-specific delayed complication: Erosion of the tube through overlying conjunctiva

3249. MC form of choroidal effusion after glaucoma surgery: Serous choroidal detachment

3250. MC cause of failure to identify Schlemm's canal in NPGS: Inadequate deep dissection

3251. MC mode of treatment in congenital glaucoma: Goniotomy and trabeculotomy

3252. MC complication of gonioplasty: Mild iritis

Corneal Surgery

3253. MC used scleral ring for scleral fixation: Flieringa ring

3254. MC indication of Flieringa ring:

    I.   Paediatric grafting

    II.   Aphakic PK

    III.   Open-sky extracapsular cataract extraction

3255. MC used size of Scleral fixating Flieringa rings: 17 mm and 18 mm size

3256. MC used ophthalmic suture for closing limbal and corneal wounds: Nylon 10-0

3257. MC indication for IOL exchange with concurrent penetrating keratoplasty: Corneal edema secondary to pseudophakic bullous keratopathy (PBK)

3258. MC used Glaucoma Drainage Implant (GDI) Devices:

    I.   Ahmed Glaucoma Valve (AGV), model FP7

    II.   Baerveldt Glaucoma Implant (BGI), model 101–350

3259. MC complication of GDI Devices: Conjunctival erosion over GDI

3260. MC site of GDI Implantation: Superotemporal quadrant

3261. MC cause of failure of a GDI in controlling IOP: Excessive fibrosis around the explant

3262. MC use of limbal autografts: Pterygium surgery

3263. MC postoperative complication of LR-CLAL (Living-Related Conjunctival–Limbal Allograft) Transplant: Acute rejection (25-33%)

3264. MC corneal wound complication: Wound dehiscence

Retina & Vitreous Surgery

3265. MC retinal procedure: Intravitreal injections

3266. MC complication of intravitreal injection: Subconjunctival haemorrhage (SCH) (aka Hyposphagma)

3267. MC utilized suture materials for scleral buckle:
    I.   5-0 nonabsorbable nylon suture
    II. 5-0 nonabsorbable soft suture such as polyester Mersilene

3268. MC used surgical approach to vitrectomy:
    I.   Closed technique (Charles, MC used now)
    II. Open sky technique (Hirose, rarely used now)

3269. MC complication in the postoperative course of ERM removal surgery: Cataract formation (not related to epimacular membrane or ILM removal but to vitrectomy itself)

3270. MC intraoperative complication of MH surgery: Iatrogenic retinal break

3271. MC indication for pars plana lensectomy: Crystalline lens or lens fragment dislocation into the vitreous cavity as a complication of cataract extraction

3272. MC complication of endoresection of choroidal melanoma:
    I. Uncontrolled haemorrhage
    II. Incomplete tumor resection
    III. Lens touch
    IV. Entry-site tears

3273. MC complication following vitrectomy: Development of cataract

3274. MC cause of sticky silicone oil in SOR surgery: Residual vitreous cortex in the area of adhesion (patches of silicone oil that are firmly attached to the retina and cannot be removed with suction alone)

3275. MC performed operation in modern vitreoretinal practice: Pars Plana Vitrectomy

3276. MC form of PVR in retinal dialysis: Subretinal bands

3277. MC used site for intravitreal injection: Inferotemporal quadrant

3278. MC complication of macular hole surgery: Progression of nuclear sclerotic cataract

3279. MC replacement material for the vitreous:

   I.   BSS

   II. Silicone oil

3280. MC retinal vascular obstruction after retrobular anaesthesia: CRAO

3281. MC use of viscoelastic agents by the vitreoretinal surgeon: As an optical-binding substance between the corneal contact lens and the corneal surface

3282. MC approach that mostly decides the time that vitrectomy should be undertaken in endophthalmitis:

   I.   Worsening despite a proper intravitreal injection

   II. Lack of response to two repeat intravitreal injections

3283. MC application of macular translocation: Management of recent-onset subfoveal CNV

3284. MC serious complication of limited macular translocation: Rhegmatogenous retinal detachment (RRD) (7.8–42.8%)

3285. MC complication of submacular surgery: Recurrent CNV

3286. MC cause of hypotony maculopathy: Glaucoma filtration surgery

3287. MC indication for diabetic vitrectomy:

    I.   Nonclearing Vitreous haemorrhage

    II.   Tractional retinal detachment

    III.   Refractory diabetic macular edema

    IV.   Combined tractional and rhegmatogenous retinal detachment

    V.   High risk PDR with anterior segment neovascularization and opaque media, severe premacular subhyaloid haemorrhage, vitreopapillary traction, ghost-cell glaucoma

3288. MC intraoperative complication during diabetic vitrectomy: Corneal epithelial haze

3289. MC postoperative complication of diabetic vitrectomy: Cataract formation

3290. MC intraoperative complications of vitrectomy surgery:

    I.   Iatrogenic breaks (6%)

    II.   Lens damage in phakic eyes (3%)

3291. MC location of iatrogenic holes in vitrectomy surgery: Close to the sclerotomies

3292. MC cause of detachment requiring reoperation following pneumatic retinopexy: Development of a new retinal break with new rather than persistent retinal detachment

MOST COMMONS IN OPHTHALMOLOGY

3293. MC indications for intraocular gas injection:

   I. Retinal detachment surgery with vitrectomy

   II. Pneumatic retinopexy

   III. Retinal detachment surgery with scleral buckle

   IV. Macular hole surgery

   V. Displacement of subretinal haemorrhage

   VI. Postvitrectomy gas exchange in vitrectomized eyes

3294. MC used gases with Pneumatic Retinopexy (PR):

   I. Sulphur hexafluoride (SF6)

   II. Perfluoropropane (C3F8)

3295. MC content of silicone oil used in VR surgeries: Polydimethylsiloxane (PDMS)

3296. MC indication for the use of silicone oil: Retinal detachment with severe PVR

3297. MC use of Prophylactic scleral buckling: To treat progressive subclinical detachments

3298. MC form of retinectomy: Removal of the anterior flap of a horseshoe tear

3299. MC indication for a relaxing retinotomy: PVR (particularly anterior PVR)

3300. MC used short-term intraoperative instrument for internal tamponade of the vitreous cavity: Perfluorocarbon liquid (PFCL)

3301. MC indications for the use of PFCL in vitrectomy:
   I.   Treatment of complex detachments
   II. PVR
   III. Giant tears

3302. MC cause of open angle glaucoma after buckling surgery: Steroid response

3303. MC cause of visual loss after successful scleral buckling: Epiretinal membranes

3304. MC presentation of PVR: Epiretinal proliferation causing traction on the retina in an eye with a RRD

3305. MC late complication of VR surgery for Proliferative vitreoretinopathy (PVR): Regrowth of surface retinal membranes leading to retinal detachment and tractional retinal tears

3306. MC type of retinal detachment recurrence after PVR surgery: Inferior recurrence of retinal detachment with or without a new or reopened retinal break inferiorly in association with light SO

3307. MC postoperative complications after vitrectomy for diabetic retinopathy:

   I. Elevated intraocular pressure

   II. Corneal erosion

   III. Fibrin formation

   IV. Bleeding

   V. Retinal detachment

3308. MC severe postoperative complication following vitrectomy for diabetic retinopathy:

   I. Anterior hyaloidal fibrovascular proliferation (AHFP)

   II. Neovascular glaucoma (previously most common)

3309. MC side effects of Intravitreal triamcinolone acetate (IVTA): Steroid-induced elevation of intraocular pressure

3310. MC complication of SRF (Subretinal Fluid) Drainage: Hypotony

3311. MC complication following epiretinal membrane (ERM) surgery: Formation or progression of cataract

3312. MC source of detachment following epiretinal membrane (ERM) surgery: Unidentified entry site breaks at the time of surgery

3313. MC illumination method used during vitrectomy surgery: Direct endoillumination probe

3314. MC cause of diffuse haze or black spots in endoscopic view in vitrectomy: Build-up of remnant of powder from the gloves of the surgery team

3315. MC complication associated with IOLs during vitrectomy: Difficult visualization especially when working in an air-filled eye

3316. MC postoperative complication in PDR patients: Vitreous Haemorrhage

3317. MC used vitrectomy systems by surgeons worldwide: 23-gauge instrument vitrectomy (developed by Eckart)

3318. MC corneal complication during vitrectomy surgery:
   I. Epithelial defects
   II. Epithelial corneal edema
   III. Descemet membrane-endothelium folds

3319. MC cause of persistent restriction of eye movements after retinal detachment surgery: Fat adherence and periocular scarring

Oculoplastic Surgery

3320. MC used procedure to correct an involutional entropion with a 'spastic' component: Horizontal (transverse) lid split and everting sutures

3321. MC used Posterior lamellar flaps: Tarso-conjunctival flap from the upper lid for reconstruction of lower lid defects (Landolt–Hughes tarso-conjunctival flap)

3322. MC complication of transconjunctival blepharoplasty: Inadequate fat excision

3323. MC cause of failed DCR:
    I.   Mucosal scarring across the ostium (membranous scarring)
    II. Sump syndrome
    III. Inadequate bony removal

3324. MC cause of failure of laser DCR: Stenosis of the rhinostomy

3325. MC used tube for Conjunctivodacryocystorhinostomy (CDCR): Pyrex glass tube

3326. MC indication for endoscopic Conjunctivodacryocystorhinostomy (CDCR): Canalicular blockage

3327. MC complication of endoscopic DCR: Excessive bleeding

3328. MC treatment for lateral orbital rhytids (Crow's feet): Botulinum toxin type A (BoNTA)

3329. MC performed two stage eyelid sharing procedure: Cutler Beard

3330. MC performed transconjunctival orbitotomies:
- I. Medial transconjunctival anterior orbitotomy
- II. Medial transcaruncular incision
- III. Lower eyelid transconjunctival approach

3331. MC procedure performed for involutional entropion: Lateral tarsal strip

3332. MC performed procedure for horizontal lower lid laxity: Tarsal strip procedure

3333. MC cause for recurrence following a tarsal strip procedure: Failure to address cicatricial eyelid changes

3334. MC setting in which patients require exenteration: Secondary orbital tumors

3335. MC origin of secondary orbital tumors: Maxillary sinus

3336. MC tumors requiring exenteration due to significant orbital invasion:
- I. BCC
- II. SCC
- III. Melanoma

MOST COMMONS IN OPHTHALMOLOGY

3337. MC indication for orbital decompression: Graves' ophthalmopathy

3338. MC significant complication of orbital decompression for graves' ophthalmopathy: Diplopia

3339. MC surgical approach used for orbital decompression: Antero ethmoidal decompression

3340. MC surgical incision used for orbital fat decompression:
   I. Transconjunctival lower lid incision
   II. Upper lid crease incision

3341. MC type of Temporary Suture Tarsorrhaphy: Partial lateral tarsorrhaphy

3342. MC reported side effect following Botox ptosis: Superior rectus underaction (68-80%)

3343. MC principles of surgical repair of ectropion: Tightening or shortening procedures centrally, laterally or medially

3344. MC indication of upper eyelid blepharoplasty: Functional > Cosmetic

3345. MC indication of lower eyelid blepharoplasty: Cosmetic > Functional

3346. MC postoperative complication of lower eyelid blepharoplasty: Ectropion and retraction

3347. MC cause of lower lid ectropion after blepharoplasty: Failure to recognize a lax lower lid before surgery

3348. MC surgical approaches described in lower lid blepharoplasty are:

    I.   Transconjunctival

    II.   Skin–muscle flap blepharoplasty

3349. MC complication of epicanthoplasty: Formation of hypertrophic Scar

3350. MC damaged muscle in blepharoplasty surgery: Inferior oblique muscle (as it is the most anterior muscle in the orbit)

3351. MC indication for external ethmoidectomy and medial orbital decompression: Compressive optic neuropathy caused by an enlarged medial rectus muscle in patients with dysthyroid orbitopathy

3352. MC aesthetic problem following endoscopic browlift: Inadequate elevation of one or both brows

3353. MC complication in lower eyelid recession: Undercorrection

3354. MC complication in upper eyelid recession:

    I.   Overcorrection

    II.   Undercorrection

3355. MC determining factors in the choice of surgical procedure for ptosis repair: Amount and type of ptosis and the degree of levator function

3356. MC procedures used for ptosis repair:

    I.   External levator resection

II. Müller's muscle conjunctival resection (MMCR)

III. Frontalis sling

IV. Full-thickness horizontal eyelid resection

3357. MC complication of Muller's Muscle–Conjunctival Resection (MMCR) for ptosis: Undercorrection

3358. MC procedure used to correct ptosis with poor levator function regardless of the etiology: Frontalis sling procedure

3359. MC non-surgical method of ptosis repair: Mechanical lifting of the upper lid by tape, skin adhesives, and lid crutches

3360. MC postoperative complication of ptosis repair:

   I. Undercorrection > overcorrection

   II. Asymmetry of the eyelid fold and crease

3361. MC intraoperative complication in ptosis surgery: Haemorrhage

3362. MC complication from posterior eyelid ptosis repair: Corneal irritation

3363. MC eyelid surgery performed today: Upper lid blepharoplasty

3364. MC concomitant structural deficiencies that require correction at the time of blepharoplasty:

   I. Brow ptosis

   II. Blepharoptosis with levator aponeurotic disinsertion

III. Lateral canthal and lid margin laxity

3365. MC cause of diplopia after upper lid blepharoplasty: Dysfunction of the superior oblique complex

3366. MC complication after open brow lifting: Paraesthesia

3367. MC complaint after endoscopic brow lifting: Postoperative numbness of the anterior scalp and forehead

3368. MC indications for Mohs micrographic surgery (MMS):
   I. Basal Cell Carcinoma (BCC)
   II. Squamous Cell Carcinoma (SCC)

3369. MC cause of local recurrence after Mohs micrographic surgery (MMS): Technical errors

3370. MC neurosurgical approach for the microsurgical clipping of intracranial aneurysms: Pterional craniotomy

3371. MC used needles in ophthalmic plastic surgery: Reverse cutting needles

3372. MC site for recurrence of brow ptosis postoperatively: Lateral eyebrow

3373. MC type of cautery used in ophthalmic plastic surgery: Bovie type (monopolar)

3374. MC injured nerve during facelift surgery: The greater auricular nerve (7% of patients)

3375. MC major complication after facelift surgery: Hematoma formation

3376. MC condition requiring punctoplasty: Punctal stenosis

3377. MC approach used for lateral orbitotomy: Stallard-Wright's procedure

3378. MC indication of lateral orbitotomy: Intraconal processes for complete removal

3379. MC repair technique of Upper eyelid defects involving greater than 50% of the lid margin: Cutler-Beard procedure

3380. MC repair technique of Moderate Defects Involving the Lower Eyelid Margin: Modified superior Tenzel semicircular rotation flap in conjunction with an inferior cantholysis

3381. MC monocanalicular stent used: Mini Monoka (FCI Ophthalmics)

3382. MC principles of surgical repair of entropion: Everting sutures, transverse lid split, retractor plication and horizontal shortening

3383. MC used free-graft sources for the eyelids:
   I. Upper eyelid skin from the normal contralateral lid (if present)
   II. Retroauricular skin
   III. Supraclavicular and infraclavicular skin
   IV. Upper inner arm (volar surface) skin
   V. Inner thigh skin

3384. MC technique for large full thickness reconstruction of the lower eyelid:

   I.   Modified Hughes tarsoconjunctival flap

   II. Hewes laterally based tarsoconjunctival flap

   III. Mustarde flap

3385. MC technique used for large, full thickness upper eyelid reconstruction:

   I.   Cutler-Beard procedure

   II. Glabellar flap

   III. Laterally based transposition flap from the suprabrow area

3386. MC type of flaps used for eyelid reconstruction:

   I.   Rectangular advancement flaps

   II. Rotation flaps

   III. Transposition flaps

3387. MC used flap for moderate lower eyelid reconstruction: Modified Tenzel semicircular rotation flap

3388. MC used peels for dark circles:

   I.   Trichloroacetic acid (TCA)

   II. Phenol peels

3389. MC used materials for alloplastic facial implants:

   I.   Solid silicone

MOST COMMONS IN OPHTHALMOLOGY

    II.   Expanded polytetrafluoroethylene

3390. MC used facial filler material: Hyaluronic Acid filler (Restylane)

3391. MC area of face treated with facial fillers: Lower face

3392. MC site for Non-animal source hyaluronic acid (NASHA) injection: Nasolabial folds

3393. MC used ablative resurfacing lasers in periocular region:
    I.   Ultrapulsed CO2 laser
    II.   Erbium: Yttrium-aluminium-garnet (YAG) laser

3394. MC areas of recurrent post-laser rhytids:
    I.   Glabellar furrows
    II.   Periocular and perioral rhytids

3395. MC adverse effect of Biosynthetic polymer filler "Sculptra" (Poly-L-lactic acid): Nodule formation

3396. MC performed treatment for paralytic lagophthalmos: Placement of a weight in the upper eyelid

3397. MC performed Rhytidectomy procedures:
    I.   Vintage (subcutaneous) rhytidectomy
    II.   Rhytidectomy with superficial elevation and refixation of the superficial musculoaponeurotic system (SMAS)

III. Deep plane rhytidectomy

Strabismus Surgery

3398. MC used weakening procedure in strabismus surgery: Recessions

3399. MC used strengthening procedure in strabismus surgery: Resections

3400. MC indication for extraocular muscle surgery in adults: Elimination or reduction of diplopia or asthenopia

3401. MC indication of Harada-Ito procedure: Bilateral superior oblique palsies when there is no or only a minimal vertical deviation in primary position

3402. MC indication of Full Tendon transposition: Lateral rectus muscle palsy

3403. MC indication for adjustable sutures in squint surgery:

   I. Squint resurgery
   II. Paretic or restrictive disease

3404. MC complication occurring after a botulinum toxin injection of an extraocular muscle: Transient blepharoptosis

3405. MC transient EOM paralysis after BOTOX to EOM: Inferior rectus muscle since gravity causes excess botulinum toxin to settle to the bottom of the orbit

3406. MC lost muscle during strabismus surgery: Medial rectus (usually during recession surgery, other three rectus muscles are rarely lost because of their connection to the oblique muscles)

3407. MC performed operation to correct infantile esotropia: Recession of both medial rectus muscles

3408. MC complication of surgery for congenital esotropia: Unsatisfactory alignment

3409. MC complication of surgery for partially accommodative esotropia: Unsatisfactory alignment

3410. MC indication of Bilateral medial rectus recession: Correction of nonaccommodative esotropia

3411. MC complication of surgery for nonaccommodative esotropia: Unsatisfactory alignment

3412. MC indication for superior oblique muscle strengthening: Congenital superior oblique muscle palsy

3413. MC performed superior oblique muscle strengthening procedure: Superior oblique tendon tuck

3414. MC performed superior oblique weakening procedure:
   I. Superior oblique tenotomy and tenectomy
   II. Wright silicone tendon expander

3415. MC indication for Superior oblique weakening procedures:
   I. To treat Brown's syndrome
   II. A-pattern strabismus associated with bilateral superior oblique overaction
   III. Unilateral superior oblique muscle overaction

3416. MC complication following superior oblique tuck: Iatrogenic Brown syndrome

3417. MC indication for surgical correction in Congenital Brown's syndrome or chronic acquired Brown's syndrome:
   I. Chin-up head posture
   II. Face turn away from the affected eye

3418. MC adverse results of the surgical treatment of true Brown's syndrome:
   I. Under-corrections or over-corrections
   II. Iatrogenic superior oblique palsy

MOST COMMONS IN OPHTHALMOLOGY

3419. MC used anaesthesia for strabismus surgery: General anaesthesia

3420. MC complication of adjustable suture strabismus surgery: Excessive postoperative discomfort from exposed sutures

3421. MC done torsional strabismus procedure: Harada-Ito procedure on the superior oblique tendon

3422. MC surgical procedure for pseudodivergence excess exotropia: Symmetric recession of both lateral rectus muscles

3423. MC complication of strabismus surgery: Globe perforation (Incidence of 1:1000, 0.13% to 1% of cases)

3424. MC suture used for strabismus surgery: Vicryl (Ethicon)

Misc Surgery

3425. MC source of postoperative infection: Patient

3426. MC application of telemicroscopes: Surgical loupes

3427. MC approach of facial nerve block in which permanent facial palsy may result: Nadbath approach

MOST COMMONS IN OPHTHALMOLOGY

3428. MC topical anesthetic agents for topical anaesthesia in intra-ocular surgery: Proparacaine

3429. MC arrhythmia in general anaesthesia: Sudden onset of atrial fibrillation

3430. MC complication of retrobulbar block: Retrobulbar haemorrhage

3431. MC cause of cancellation on the day of surgery in the elderly patient with eye disease: Arrhythmias

3432. MC complication with peribulbar anaesthesia: Subconjunctival haemorrhage

3433. MC agent used for sterilisation of operating room: Formaldehyde

3434. MC used fibrin glue products:

    I.   Tisseel/Tissucol Fibrin Sealant (Baxter Immuno)

    II.   Evicel (Johnson & Johnson) Fibrin Sealant

    III.   Vitagel (Orthovita) Surgical Hemostat

    IV.   ReliSeal (Reliance Life Sciences)

3435. MC laser used for laser suture lysis: Argon laser (500 mW for 0.05 second and 100μm spot)

3436. MC method of preservation of Amniotic Membrane: Freezing

3437. MC use of amniotic membrane grafts: Ocular surface reconstruction

3438. MC surgical procedure used for Trigeminal Neuralgia:

I. Microvascular decompression

II. Percutaneous radiofrequency thermocoagulation of the ganglion

3439. MC quadrant chosen for Posterior Subtenon (PST) Injection:

Superotemporal

MOST COMMONS IN OPHTHALMOLOGY

Trauma & Emergencies

General Eye Trauma

3440. MC cause for attendance at an eye hospital emergency department: An injury to the eye or its surrounding tissues

3441. MC ophthalmic indication for hospitalization: Eye trauma

3442. MC reason for extended hospitalization of ophthalmologic patients: Eye trauma

3443. MC cause of unilateral blindness in children: Eye trauma

3444. MC form of ophthalmic trauma:

    I.   Corneal abrasions

    II.   Corneal foreign bodies

3445. MC circumstances in which ocular injury occurs:

    I.   Domestic accidents (40%)

    II.   Industrials (13%)

    III.   Street/highway accidents (13%)

3446. MC sources of eye injuries:

    I.   Blunt object (31%)

    II.   Sharp object (18%)

    III.   Motor vehicle crash (9%)

MOST COMMONS IN OPHTHALMOLOGY

3447. MC risk factors for eye injury:

    I.   Male gender (approximately 80% of open-globe injuries)

    II.   Race (Hispanics and African- Americans have higher risk)

    III.   Professional activity (e. G., military personnel)

    IV.   Younger age (third decade)

    V.   Low education

    VI.   Contact sports

    VII.   Failure to comply with safety devices and equipment

3448. MC involved ocular tissue in eye trauma: Cornea

3449. MC cause of the eye injuries during the war: Explosions with fragmentation injury

3450. MC cause of photic injury: Sun gazing

3451. MC injuries to welders: Eye injuries

3452. MC source of eye injuries to welders: Molten and cold metal particles striking the eye

3453. MC location of conjunctival foreign bodies: Sulcus subtarsalis in upper palpebral conjunctiva

3454. MC object to be found as conjunctival foreign body: Wing of an insect

3455. MC organisms cultured from infected dog bite wounds:

MOST COMMONS IN OPHTHALMOLOGY

  I. Pasteurella multicida
  II. Pasteurella canis
  III. Streptococci species
  IV. Staphylococci species

3456. MC isolates from human bite wounds:

  I. Staphylococcus aureus
  II. Group A beta-hemolytic Streptococcus
  III. Eikenella corrodens

3457. MC type of injury caused by airbag deployment: Corneal abrasion

3458. MC type of retinal injuries by airbag deployment: Retinal breaks at vitreous base

Open & Close Globe Injury

3459. MC injured corneal tissue in blunt trauma:

  I. Epithelium
  II. Endothelium

3460. MC site of ruptured globe in blunt trauma: Just behind rectus muscle insertion

3461. MC location of retinal breaks in blunt ocular trauma:

  I. SuperoNasal quadrant

II. InferoTemporal quadrant

3462. MC location of retinal tears in open globe injuries:

   I. Just posterior to the scleral wound

   II. 180° away from scleral wound (caused by direct traction)

3463. MC cause of early IOP rise in blunt trauma: Tears in the trabecular meshwork

3464. MC retinal break produced by the blunt trauma: Retinal dialysis

3465. MC cause of late onset retinal detachment in blunt trauma: Retinal dialysis

3466. MC location of posttraumatic retinal dialysis:

   I. Inferotemporal (27-73%)

   II. Superonasal (2-46%)

   III. Superotemporal

   IV. Inferonasal

3467. MC type of trauma causing retinal dialysis: Blow from the fist

3468. MC cause of traumatic retinal detachment: Blunt trauma

3469. MC cause of severe eye injuries in the world today: Sports

3470. MC cause of acquired iris deficiency: Trauma (approx. 35% of our cases of iris deficiency)

3471. MC cause of zonular insufficiency: Trauma

3472. MC UBM findings in closed globe injury:

    I.   Zonular deficiency (64.2%)

    II.   Angle recession (43.3%)

    III.   Iridodialysis (17.9%)

    IV.   Dislocated lens (16.4%)

    V.   Hyphema in 13.4%

    VI.   Peripheral anterior synechiae (8.9%)

3473. MC UBM findings in open globe injury:

    I.   Zonular deficiency (54.8%)

    II.   Iridodialysis (26.2%)

    III.   Peripheral anterior synechiae (26.2%)

    IV.   Angle recession (14.3%)

    V.   Ruptured anterior capsule (14.3%)

3474. MC sign of postcontusional eye injury: Angle recession

3475. MC type of traumatic glaucoma: Angle recession glaucoma

3476. MC vision limiting factor in open globe injury: Traumatic cataract

3477. MC site of bleeding in traumatic hyphema: A tear at the anterior aspect of the ciliary body (70% of cases)

3478. MC risk factor for developing corneal blood staining: Hyphema combined with secondary glaucoma

3479. MC interval in which rebleeding occurs in hyphema: Day 2 to 5

3480. MC ocular cranial nerve involved in corneal trauma: 3rd Cranial nerve

3481. MC location of scleral rupture in ocular compression injury:

    I. Limbus

    II. Parallel to the muscle insertions between the insertion

    III. Equator of the globe

3482. MC cause of IOFB (Intra Ocular Foreign Body):

    I. Younger patients: Projectile weapon or explosion (60%)

    II. Adults: Hammering (84%)

3483. MC encountered IOFB material:

    I. Iron

    II. Copper

3484. MC setting leading to IOFB (Intra Ocular Foreign Body): Hammering metal on metal

3485. MC encountered organic IOFB: Wood

3486. MC cause of choroidal rupture: Contusion

3487. MC secondary complication of choroidal rupture: Development of choroidal neovascularization

3488. MC location of choroidal rupture:
- I. Posterior pole
- II. Midperipheral fundus

3489. MC pattern of choroidal rupture: Semicircular lines circumscribing the optic nerve head in the peripapillary region

3490. MC location of choroidal rupture: Temporal to the optic nerve and through the macula

3491. MC cause of litigation against the ophthalmologist in a trauma case: Missed IOFB

3492. MC site of entry of IOFB:
- I. Cornea (65%)
- II. Sclera (25%)
- III. Limbus (10%)

3493. MC patterns of iris injury after severe blunt trauma: Sphincter tears and dialysis of the iris root

3494. MC cause of poor visual outcome in vitreous haemorrhage associated with nonpenetrating trauma: Macular scar

3495. MC cause of chorioretinitis sclopetaria: When a high-velocity missile strikes or passes adjacent to but does not penetrate the globe

3496. MC quadrant involved in traumatic detachment of the vitreous base: Inferotemporal

3497. MC cause of vitreous haemorrhage in children: Trauma (Manifest & Occult)

3498. MC location of Commotio Retinae: Posterior pole (aka Berlin's edema)

Orbital Trauma

3499. MC periorbital fracture seen in ophthalmic plastic surgical practice: Blow out fractures

3500. MC fractured wall in orbital blow-in fracture:

    I. Roof

    II. Lateral wall

3501. MC fractured wall in orbital blow-out fracture:

    I. Orbital floor (67%) (posteromedial) (not the thinnest wall but most frequently fractured having no underlying support within the maxillary sinus)

    II. Combined orbital floor and medial wall (14%)

III. Medial wall (8%) (lamina papyracea, the thinnest of the orbital walls but the network of septations within the ethmoid air cells acts as a supporting scaffolding to the medial orbital wall)

IV. Orbital Roof (6%)

3502. MC fracture that presents primarily to the ophthalmologist:

I. The isolated floor fracture (blowout)

II. Zygomatico maxillary Complex (ZMC Fracture)

3503. MC presenting complaint of blowout fracture: Vertical diplopia, with limitation of up- or down-gaze (entrapment of orbital tissues in the fracture plate)

3504. MC misalignment in cases of an orbital fracture: Hypotropia from entrapment of the muscle or of orbital septae

3505. MC cause of orbital abscess: Spread of a preexisting sinus infection

3506. MC location of subperiosteal haemorrhage in orbital trauma: Orbital roof

3507. MC EOM involved in direct EOM trauma:

I. Inferior rectus

II. Medial rectus

III. Lateral rectus

IV. Superior rectus

V. Inferior oblique

VI. Superior oblique

3508. MC cause of isolated extraocular muscle damage: Trauma

3509. MC muscle involved in iatrogenic muscle trauma:

I. Inferior rectus muscle

II. Inferior oblique muscle

3510. MC form of laceration to the nasolacrimal drainage system: Canalicular laceration

3511. MC cause for canalicular laceration:

I. Blunt trauma from a fist punch (23%)

II. Dog bite (19%)

3512. MC cause of canalicular laceration in children: Dog bite

3513. MC cause of posttraumatic ptosis: Lid edema and hematoma

3514. MC orbital organic foreign body: Wood

3515. MC avulsed extraocular muscles:

I. Inferior rectus

II. Medial rectus

3516. MC form of incomitant strabismus produced by "Flap Tear" of Extraocular muscles: Hyperdeviation greatest on downgaze due to partial avulsion of the ipsilateral inferior rectus

Chemical Injury

3517. MC cause of chemical ocular injury: Sulfuric acid (usually the result of the explosion of a car battery)

3518. MC cause of storage battery explosion:

    I.   Lit matches (used to see battery cells)

    II.   Incorrect use of jumper cables

3519. MC alkalis causing the injury:

    I.   Calcium hydroxide (lime) (In form of plaster, Most common work-related chemical injury)

    II.   Ammonium hydroxide (ammonia)

    III.   Sodium hydroxide (lye)

    IV.   Potassium hydroxide (KOH, potash)

    V.   Magnesium hydroxide (Mg[OH]2)

3520. MC acids causing injury:

MOST COMMONS IN OPHTHALMOLOGY

    I.   Sulfuric acid (H_2SO_4; the most common cause, In form of automobile battery explosion)

    II.   Sulphurous acid (H_2SO_3)

    III.   Hydrofluoric (HF; rapidly penetrating and causing the most serious injuries)

    IV.   Acetic (CH_3COOH)

    V.   Chromic (Cr_2O_3)

    VI.   Hydrochloric (HCL)

3521. MC source of ammonia in alkali injury: Household ammonia (a 7% solution used as a cleaning agent)

3522. MC therapeutic mistakes in the management of severe chemical injuries of the eye:

    I.   Failure to diagnose and treat persistent limbal stem-cell dysfunction properly at an early stage

    II.   Failure to try aggressively to control ocular inflammation

3523. MC vesicant used in chemical weapons: Sulphur mustard

3524. MC cause of failure to restore vision to an alkali-injured eye: End stage glaucoma

Optic Nerve Related Trauma

3525. MC site of visual pathway trauma: Optic nerve

3526. MC form of TON (Traumatic Optic Neuropathy): Indirect TON (Posterior indirect TON is most common)

3527. MC type of injuries causing TON (Traumatic Optic Neuropathy):
    I.   Posterior indirect injuries
    II. Chiasmal injuries
    III. Direct injuries

3528. MC portion of the optic nerve damaged following closed head trauma:
    I. Intracanalicular portion of the optic nerve
    II. Intracranial portion of the optic nerve

3529. MC cause of traumatic optic neuropathy:
    I.   Deceleration injury directed to the ipsilateral forehead or to the midface region from motor vehicle and bicycle accidents (45% of the cases)
    II. Falls (27%)
    III. Motorcycle crashes (18% of the cases)

3530. MC cause of Traumatic Optic Neuropathy in Children:
    I. Falls

II. Road traffic crashes

III. Sporting injuries

3531. MC reported surgical intervention for Traumatic Optic Neuropathy (TON): Decompression of the optic canal

3532. MC indication for endoscopic optic canal decompression: Traumatic optic neuropathy (TON)

Shaken Baby Syndrome

3533. MC manifestation of Shaken baby syndrome (SBS)/Child abuse: Retinal haemorrhages

3534. MC inciting factor for child abuse in infancy: Parental frustration over the child's crying or feeding

3535. MC intracranial finding in shaken baby syndrome: Subdural hematoma

3536. MC type of child abuse resulting in death: Abusive head trauma

3537. MC perpetrators of Shaken Baby Syndrome:

I. Biological fathers

II. Biologically unrelated boyfriends of the mother

III. Babysitters

3538. MC type of Bone injury in Shaken baby syndrome: Rib fractures

3539. MC cause of permanent visual loss in child abuse: Injury to the occipital cortex

3540. MC cause of burns in Child abuse syndrome: Scalding with hot water

3541. MC sign of ocular injury: Conjunctival haemorrhage

3542. MC form of Child maltreatment:
    I. Neglect in various forms
    II. Physical abuse
    III. Sexual abuse
    IV. Emotional abuse

3543. MC cause of visual loss and blindness following SBS: Cortical visual impairment

Misc Eye Trauma

3544. MC complication of Terson syndrome: Appearance of Epiretinal membrane

3545. MC underlying cause of AION: Hypertension

MOST COMMONS IN OPHTHALMOLOGY

3546. MC radiological imaging study in patients with severe peri/ocular trauma: CT scan

3547. MC source of exogenous emphysema of conjunctiva: Explosion

3548. MC manifestation of AC structural damage: Hyphema

3549. MC cause of retinal detachment in children: Trauma

3550. MC cause of acquired oculomotor palsy: Injury (generally intracranial)

3551. MC ocular manifestation of whiplash syndrome: Horner's syndrome

3552. MC complication of eyelid margin laceration: Lid notching

3553. MC cause of failure of repair of traumatic RD: PVR

3554. MC vitreous related pathology in eye trauma: Vitreous haemorrhage

3555. MC avoidable error in contusion related eye trauma: Not to consider early surgery for vitreous haemorrhage

3556. MC preventable cause of enucleation due to phthisis: Anterior PVR

3557. MC underlying cause of Terson syndrome in adults: Subarachnoid bleeding from a cerebral aneurysm (particularly an aneurysm of the anterior communicating artery)

3558. MC military tear gas: 2-chlorobenzalmalonitrile (CS)

3559. MC affected ocular structure by siderosis:
    I. Iris

II. Lens

3560. MC pupillary abnormality in siderosis: Mid-dilated pupil that is minimally reactive to light

3561. MC clinical findings in siderosis:
   I. Iris heterochromia, with the affected eye having a rust-brown discoloration
   II. Diffuse cataract
   III. RPE degeneration affecting the peripheral retina in the early stages before progressing to the posterior pole
   IV. Vitreous opacification

3562. MC ERG finding in siderosis: Reduction in b-wave amplitudes

3563. MC affected ocular structure by chalcosis:
   I. Cornea (Descemet's membrane)
   II. Iris
   III. Lens (Anterior lens capsule)
   IV. Macula (ILM)

3564. MC clinical findings in chalcosis:
   I. The Kayser-Fleischer ring

II. Iris heterochromia with the affected eye having a greenish discoloration

III. A pathognomonic sunflower cataract

IV. Refractile precipitates in the macular region

V. Vitreous opacification

3565. MC cause of Emphysema of the orbit and eyelids: Medial wall orbital fractures

3566. MC thermal injuries to the ocular surface in childhood: Cigarette burns of the cornea (these occur in toddlers and are accidental, not manifestations of abuse)

Uveitis

General Uveitis

3567. MC form of uveitis:

    I.   Anterior Uveitis (50-60%)

    II.   Posterior uveitis (15-30%)

    III.   Intermediate uveitis

3568. MC form of uveitis in children:

    I.   JIA (41.5%)

    II.   Idiopathic uveitis (21.5%)

    III.   Pars planitis (15.3%)

    IV.   Toxoplasmosis (7.7%)

3569. MC associated systemic disease with uveitis: Sarcoidosis

3570. MC form of non-infectious uveitis: HLA-B27 associated Anterior uveitis

3571. MC ocular disease associated with uveitis: Herpes simplex keratitis

3572. MC location of iris nodules in granulomatous uveitis: Pupillary margin (Koeppe's nodule)

3573. MC type of cataract in uveitis patients: Posterior subcapsular cataract

3574. MC presentation of coccidioidomycosis: Influenza like pulmonary illness

3575. MC mode of transmission of Chagas disease:

MOST COMMONS IN OPHTHALMOLOGY

    I. Vector

    II. Blood transfusion

3576. MC manifestation of chronic Chagas disease: Chagas cardiomyopathy

3577. MC infectious cause of blindness worldwide:

    I. Trachoma

    II. Onchocerciasis

3578. MC clinical manifestation of onchocerciasis affects

    I. Skin

    II. Eye

    III. Lymphatic system

3579. MC pathology associated with loa loa infestation in humans: Calabar swellings

3580. MC ocular involvement in loiasis: Subconjunctval migration of worm

3581. MC reported corneal finding in uveitis: Keratic precipitates (KPs)

3582. MC fungal disease associated with uveitis: Histoplasmosis

3583. MC macular disease seen in uveitis: CME

3584. MC sequelae of uveitis:

    I. Posterior synechiae

    II. CME

3585. MC cause of pseudohypopyons in adults develop: Systemic lymphoma or leukemic relapse

3586. MC systemic lymphoma subtype to affect the eye: Diffuse large B-cell lymphoma (DLBCL)

Anterior Uveitis

3587. MC type of cells seen in anterior chamber in uveitis patients: T lymphocytes

3588. MC causes of Anterior uveitis:

    I.   Idiopathic nongranulomatous anterior uveitis 37.8%

    II.   Seronegative HLA-B27-associated arthropathies 21.6%

    III.   Juvenile idiopathic arthritis 10.8%

    IV.   Herpetic uveitis 9.7% (herpes simplex and herpes zoster)

    V.   Sarcoidosis 5.85%

    VI.   Fuchs' heterochromic iridocyclitis 5.0%

    VII.   Systemic lupus erythematosus 3.3%

    VIII.   Intraocular lens induced persistent uveitis 1.2%

    IX.   Posner-Schlossman syndrome 0.9%

X. Rheumatoid arthritis 0.9%

3589. MC ocular manifestations of Chikungunya virus infection: Acute anterior uveitis and retinitis

3590. MC ocular manifestation of acquired measles infection: Epithelial keratitis

3591. MC cause of infectious anterior uveitis in children: Herpes simplex and varicella zoster

3592. MC extra-articular/ocular manifestation of Ankylosing Spondylitis:
   I. Acute Anterior uveitis (AAU)
   II. Conjunctivitis

3593. MC systemic condition known to be associated with anterior uveitis in men: Ankylosing Spondylitis (17-31%)

3594. MC manifestation of Reiter syndrome:
   I. Joint involvement
   II. Ocular Involvement

3595. MC ophthalmic manifestation of Reiter syndrome:
   I. Conjunctivitis (60%)
   II. Uveitis (12%)

MOST COMMONS IN OPHTHALMOLOGY

3596. MC type of uveitis in Reiter syndrome: Nongranulomatous anterior uveitis

3597. MC pathogenesis of Reactive Arthritis: After dysentery due to gram-negative bacteria (MC Salmonella, Shigella, and Yersinia)

3598. MC cause of inflammatory oligoarthropathy in young males: Reactive Arthritis

3599. MC ocular involvement of Reactive Arthritis:
   I. Conjunctivitis (30-60%)
   II. Anterior uveitis (3-12%)

3600. MC type of scleritis in patients of Reactive Arthritis: Diffuse anterior scleritis

3601. MC joints affected by Reactive Arthritis:
   I. Knee
   II. Ankle
   III. Toe

3602. MC genitourinary problem in patients with Reactive Arthritis: Urethritis

3603. MC ocular manifestation of IBD (Inflammatory Bowel Disease):
   I. Episcleritis (29%, though it is underdiagnosed due to self-limited course)

MOST COMMONS IN OPHTHALMOLOGY

    II.   Acute nongranulomatous recurrent anterior uveitis

    III.   Scleritis

    IV.   Keratitis

3604. MC diagnosed ocular manifestation of IBD (Inflammatory Bowel Disease): Uveitis (17%)

3605. MC type of IBD associated uveitis:

    I.   Nongranulomatous, low-grade, recurrent, acute anterior uveitis (60%)

    II.   Panuveitis with associated vasculitis (30%)

    III.   Non-recurrent acute anterior uveitis (10%)

3606. MC clinical manifestation of SLE (Systemic Lupus Erythematosus): Malar Flush

3607. MC serological abnormality in SLE (Systemic Lupus Erythematosus): Elevated ANA titre

3608. MC ocular complication of SLE:

    I.   Secondary Sjogren's syndrome

    II.   Retinopathy

3609. MC retinal vascular lesions observed in patients with SLE: Cotton-wool spots (soft exudates) with and without intraretinal haemorrhages

MOST COMMONS IN OPHTHALMOLOGY

3610. MC ocular manifestation in patients with Systemic Sclerosis (SSc): Keratoconjunctivitis Sicca (KCS)

3611. MC marker antibodies for Systemic Sclerosis:
   I. Anticentromere antibodies (specific for limited SSc and found in 45–50% of these patients)
   II. Scl-70 or antitopoisomerase-1 (specific for diffuse SSc and present in 40%)

3612. MC symptom of FHI (Fuchs Heterochromatic Iridocyclitis):
   I. Floaters caused by vitreous opacities
   II. Visual deterioration caused by cataract

3613. MC histopathological finding of FHI: Iris stromal atrophy and infiltration of the iris stroma and ciliary body with lymphocytes and plasma cells

3614. MC cause of permanent vision loss in FHI patients: Glaucoma (59%)

3615. MC cause of decreased vision in FHI patients: Cataract

3616. MC form of intraocular inflammation with TINU (Tubulointerstitial Nephritis and Uveitis Syndrome): Anterior uveitis

3617. MC cause of ATIN (Acute tubulointerstitial nephritis) in adults: Drug hypersensitivity

3618. MC manifestation of HLA-B27 associated uveitis:

I. Acute iritis

   II. Retinal Vasculitis

3619. MC type of uveitis in seronegative spondyloarthropathies [SSA]:

Unilateral AAU (Acute Anterior Uveitis)

3620. MC clue for detecting Cytomegalovirus Anterior Uveitis: Unilateral, recurrent anterior uveitis without iris atrophy but with raised IOP

3621. MC uveitis types associated with raised IOP:

   I. Fuchs iridocyclitis

   II. Vogt-Koyanagi-Harada syndrome

   III. JIA-associated iridocyclitis

   IV. Iritis secondary to toxoplasmosis

3622. MC cause of elevated IOP in chronic uveitis: Open angle glaucoma

Intermediate Uveitis

3623. MC causes of intermediate uveitis:

   I. Idiopathic, 69.1%

   II. Sarcoidosis, 22.2%

   III. Multiple sclerosis, 8.0%

   IV. Lyme disease, 0.6%

MOST COMMONS IN OPHTHALMOLOGY

3624. MC form of ocular involvement by Herpes zoster ophthalmicus in AIDS patients: Keratitis

3625. MC form of ocular involvement in HZO: Iridocyclitis

3626. MC non-Langerhans cell Histiocytosis: Juvenile xanthogranuloma (JXG)

3627. MC part of body involved by Juvenile Xanthogranuloma (JXG): Skin

3628. MC extracutaneous manifestation of Juvenile Xanthogranuloma: Ocular disease

3629. MC ocular manifestations of Juvenile Xanthogranuloma: Unilateral iris lesion, spontaneous hyphaema and potentially blinding secondary glaucoma

3630. MC ocular structure involved in Juvenile Xanthogranuloma (JXG):
    I. Iris (Iris Infiltration)
    II. Choroid
    III. Orbit
    IV. Cornea

3631. MC location of skin nodule in JXG:
    I. Scalp
    II. Head & Neck

3632. MC presentation of Juvenile Xanthogranuloma (JXG): Spontaneous bleed with occurrence of a hyphema

MOST COMMONS IN OPHTHALMOLOGY

3633. MC mode of diagnosis of Juvenile Xanthogranuloma (JXG): Biopsy of skin lesion

3634. MC form of uveitis in patients with MS (Multiple Sclerosis):
   I. Idiopathic intermediate uveitis or pars planitis
   II. Granulomatous anterior uveitis

3635. MC symptom of Multiple sclerosis: Fatigue

3636. MC ocular complication of Multiple sclerosis: Atrophy of the optic nerve and inner retinal layers

3637. MC cause of severe vision loss in Intermediate uveitis or pars planitis: Cystoid macular edema

3638. MC location of snowbanks in pars planitis: Inferior retina

3639. MC causes of hypopyon uveitis:
   I. Behçet's disease
   II. Infections

3640. MC cause of sectoral iris atrophy:
   I. Herpes zoster uveitis
   II. Herpes simplex uveitis
   III. CMV uveitis

3641. MC ocular manifestation of Tick borne relapsing fever: Iritis

Posterior Uveitis

3642. MC causes of posterior uveitis:

    I.   Toxoplasmosis, 24.6%

    II.   Idiopathic, 12.3%

    III.   Cytomegalovirus retinitis, 11.6%

    IV.   Systemic lupus erythematosus, 7.9%

    V.   Birdshot retinochoroidopathy, 7.9%

    VI.   Sarcoidosis, 7.5%

    VII.   Acute retinal necrosis syndrome, 5.5%

    VIII.   Epstein-Barr virus retinochoroiditis, 2.9%

    IX.   Toxocariasis, 2.5%

    X.   Adamantiades-behçet's disease (ABD), 2.0%

    XI.   Syphilis, 2.0%

    XII.   APMPPE, 2.0%

    XIII.   Serpiginous choroidopathy, 1.65%

3643. MC cause of infectious posterior uveitis in children: Toxoplasmosis

3644. MC cause of infectious posterior uveitis in immunocompetent individuals: Toxoplasmosis

MOST COMMONS IN OPHTHALMOLOGY

3645. MC cause of infectious posterior uveitis in immunocompromised individuals: Cytomegalovirus (CMV)

3646. MC ocular manifestation of Tuberculosis: Chronic granulomatous iridocyclitis that is usually bilateral

3647. MC posterior uveitis in tuberculosis:
   I. Bilateral multifocal choroiditis, with or without overlying retinal necrosis
   II. Single tubercle (focal choroiditis)

3648. MC cause of treatment failure in pulmonary TB: Nonadherence to therapy

3649. MC source of infection of leptospirosis: Urine of infected animals

3650. MC sign of ocular leptospirosis: Circumcorneal Conjunctival vasodilatation with hyperemia or haemorrhage

3651. MC form of uveitis in leptospirosis: Anterior uveitis

3652. MC ocular manifestation of brucellosis: Uveitis

3653. MC cause of death in brucellosis: Endocarditis

3654. MC used test for brucellosis: SAT (Serum Agglutination Test)

3655. MC manifestation of leprosy: Brow hair loss and loss of lashes (Madarosis)

MOST COMMONS IN OPHTHALMOLOGY

3656. MC intraocular manifestations of leprosy: Acute and/or chronic uveitis

3657. MC cause of ARN (Acute Retinal Necrosis):

   I. Varicella–zoster virus (46%)

   II. Herpes simplex virus type 1 (25%)

   III. Herpes simplex virus type 2 (21%)

   IV. Cytomegalovirus

3658. MC cause of PORN (progressive outer retinal necrosis) : VZV infection

3659. MC manifestation of CMV ocular infection: CMV retinitis

3660. MC cause of blindness in AIDS patients: CMV retinitis

3661. MC congenital viral infection: CMV

3662. MC ocular manifestation of WNV infection (West Nile Virus): Multifocal chorioretinitis (MFC)

3663. MC ocular manifestation of RVF (Rift Valley Fever) virus infection: Bilateral macular and paramacular exudative-like lesions with retinal edema and haemorrhage

3664. MC constituents of CNVM in POHS: Vascular endothelium and RPE

3665. MC etiologic agent for mucosal leishmaniasis: L. braziliensis

3666. MC ocular abnormality seen in visceral leishmaniasis: Intraretinal haemorrhage

3667. MC ocular manifestation of cryptococcosis: Papilledema

3668. MC presentation of leukemic retinopathy: Intraretinal haemorrhages at posterior pole

3669. MC ocular finding in PAN (Poly Arteritis Nodosa): Choroidal and retinal vasculitis

3670. MC etiologic virus causing PAN: Hepatitis B

3671. MC body system involved in Wegener's Granulomatosis (WG): Upper/Lower respiratory system

3672. MC dermatologic finding in Wegener's Granulomatosis: Purpura

3673. MC presenting feature of ocular Wegener's granulomatosis: Painful proptosis with eyelid and conjunctival edema and ocular motility disturbance

3674. MC renal lesion in patients with Wegener's granulomatosis: Focal necrotizing glomerulonephritis

3675. MC neurological finding in Wegener's granulomatosis: Peripheral neuropathy

3676. MC clinical feature of polychondritis:
    I.   Auricular involvement
    II.   Arthritis

MOST COMMONS IN OPHTHALMOLOGY

3677. MC ocular manifestation of polychondritis:

   I. Episcleritis (39%)

   II. Scleritis (14%)

   III. Iridocyclitis (9%)

3678. MC cause of death in polychondritis: Pulmonary infection

3679. MC structural complication of BSRC (Birdshot Retinochoroiditis):

   Macular edema

3680. MC neurologic complaint in VKH (Vogt-Koyanagi-Harada) Syndrome:

   Headache

3681. MC visual field defect in MCP (Multifocal choroiditis with Panuveitis):

   Acute symptomatic enlargement of the blind spot in the absence of disc edema

3682. MC cause of incident visual loss in MCP (Multifocal choroiditis with panuveitis): Choroidal neovascular membranes (CNVM)

3683. MC form of vision loss in AZZOR (Acute Zonal Occult Outer Retinopathy) : Scotomas

3684. MC visual field defect in AZOOR: Blind spot enlargement with or without central scotoma

3685. MC autoimmune disease associated with AZOOR:

I. Hashimoto's thyroiditis (12%)

II. Fibromyalgia (10%)

III. Multiple sclerosis (8%)

IV. Hypothyroidism (4%)

3686. MC steroid sparing agent used for retinal vasculitis: Low dose cyclosporine

3687. MC ocular manifestation of Vogt-Koyanagi-Harada disease: Bilateral granulomatous panuveitis with exudative retinal detachments

3688. MC systemic finding of Lymphocytic choriomeningitis virus (LCMV) congenital infection: Macrocephaly and Microcephaly

3689. MC ocular finding of Lymphocytic choriomeningitis virus (LCMV) congenital infection: Chorioretinitis with peripheral or macular chorioretinal scarring

3690. MC complaints of patients with inflammation of the vitreous, retina, and choroid

I. Floaters

II. Reduced vision

3691. MC cause of Diffuse Unilateral Subacute Neuroretinitis (DUSN): Larva of ascaridoid nematodes including Toxocara canis and the dog hookworm Ancylostoma caninum

3692. MC surgical procedure leading to sympathetic ophthalmia:
   I.   Cataract extraction (particularly when complicated)
   II. Iris surgery (including iridectomy)
   III. Retinal detachment repair
   IV. Vitreoretinal surgery

3693. MC cause of sympathetic ophthalmia: Penetrating eye trauma

3694. MC duration of development of sympathetic ophthalmia: Within 3 months of original injury (70%)

3695. MC location of Serpiginous choroiditis (SC): Close to the optic disc with peripapillary lesions and fingerlike projections extending outward

3696. MC antigen used to induce Experimental autoimmune uveoretinitis (EAU): S-antigen (48-kDa protein also referred to as arrestin)

3697. MC presentation of ocular Whipple's disease: Vitritis (Uveitis)

3698. MC diagnosis confused with Multiple Evanescent White Dot Syndrome (MEWDS):

MOST COMMONS IN OPHTHALMOLOGY

I. Acute posterior multifocal placoid pigment epitheliopathy (APMPPE)

II. Birdshot retinochoroidopathy

III. Multifocal choroiditis

IV. Retinal pigment epitheliopathy

3699. MC diagnosis confused with Acute Posterior Multifocal Placoid Pigment Epitheliopathy (APMPPE):

I. Serpiginous choroiditis

II. Multiple evanescent white dot syndrome (MEWDS)

III. Birdshot choroidopathy

IV. Diffuse metastatic cancerous lesions

V. Non-Hodgkin's lymphoma

VI. Pneumocystis choroiditis

3700. MC visual field defect seen in Multiple Evanescent White Dot Syndrome (MEWDS): Enlarged Blind Spot

3701. MC differentials in case of multifocal choroiditis:

I. Histoplasmosis

II. Sarcoidosis

3702. MC differential for cases of serpiginous choroiditis: With Acute Posterior Multifocal Placoid Pigment Epitheliopathy (APMPPE)

3703. MC indication for PCR diagnostics in posterior segment uveitis: To differentiate between viral retinitis and ocular toxoplasmosis

Panuveitis

3704. MC causes of panuveitis:

    I. Idiopathic, 22.2%

    II. Sarcoidosis, 14.1%

    III. Multifocal choroiditis and panuveitis, 12.1%

    IV. Adamantiades-behçet's disease ABD, 11.6%

    V. Systemic lupus erythematosus, 9.1%

    VI. Syphilis, 5.5%

    VII. Vogt-koyanagi-harada syndrome, 5.5%

    VIII. Hla-b27 associated, 4.5%

    IX. Sympathetic ophthalmia, 4.0%

    X. Tuberculosis, 2.0%

    XI. Fungal retinitis, 2.0%

3705. MC ocular presentation of Familial juvenile systemic granulomatosis (Blau syndrome): Chronic panuveitis associated with multifocal choroiditis

Childhood Uveitis

3706. MC disease associated with childhood anterior uveitis: Juvenile Idiopathic Arthritis (JIA)

3707. MC type of JIA seen with uveitis: Oligoarticular with positive serology for antinuclear antibodies (ANA)

3708. MC ocular finding in JIA: Nongranulomatous iridocyclitis

3709. MC rheumatic disease occurring in childhood: Juvenile idiopathic arthritis (JIA)

3710. MC form of JIA: Polyarticular (30%, though uveitis occur in only 5%)

3711. MC complication in children with uveitis:
   I. Posterior synechiae
   II. Band keratopathy
   III. Cataract
   IV. Glaucoma
   V. CME
   VI. Hypotony

Behcet's Disease

3712. MC geographic location for Bechet's disease: Mediterranean countries, the Middle East, and the Far East especially Japan

3713. MC joint affected in arthritis of Bechet's disease: Knee

3714. MC finding/manifestation in Bechet's disease: Oral aphthous ulcers (96%)

3715. MC neuro-ophthalmic finding in Bechet's disease:
    I.   Optic disc hyperemia
    II. Optic atrophy

3716. MC fluorescein angiography findings of Bechet's disease:
    I.   Diffuse vascular leakage
    II. Hyperfluorescence of the optic disk
    III. Hyperfluorescence of the macula

3717. MC posterior segment finding in Bechet's disease: Retinal vasculitis (intensive retinal edema, yellowish-white exudates and haemorrhages)

3718. MC genetic marker of Behcet's disease: HLA-B51 (HLA-B5101 is MC suballele)

3719. MC indication for IFN-α in ophthalmology: Ocular involvement due to Behcet's disease (BD)

3720. MC used immunosuppressive agent for ocular Bechet's disease:

Cyclosporin A (3–5 mg/kg/day)

3721. MC part of brain involved by vascular thrombosis in Bechet's disease:

Basal ganglia and brainstem

3722. MC site of venous thrombosis in Behcet's Disease:
- I. Superior or inferior vena cava
- II. Femoral veins
- III. Cerebral veins

3723. MC cardiac manifestation of Behcet's Disease:
- I. Pericarditis
- II. Coronary vasculitis

3724. MC urogenital manifestation of Behcet's Disease: Epididymitis (4-31%)

Sarcoidosis

3725. MC associated systemic disease with uveitis: Sarcoidosis

3726. MC extrathoracic involvement of sarcoidosis: Ophthalmic (25% patients, uveitis MC)

3727. MC sight-threatening consequence of sarcoid uveitis: Macular edema

3728. MC thoracic manifestation of Sarcoidosis: Symmetrical hilar adenopathy

MOST COMMONS IN OPHTHALMOLOGY

3729. MC form of neurologic involvement in Sarcoidosis: Cranial Nerve Involvement

3730. MC cranial nerve involved in sarcoidosis:

   I. Facial nerve

   II. Optic nerve

3731. MC ocular motor nerve involved in sarcoidosis: Abducens nerve

3732. MC intracranial manifestation of sarcoidosis: Granulomatous meningitis

3733. MC manifestation of ocular sarcoidosis: Bilateral, recurrent, anterior granulomatous uveitis

3734. MC posterior segment manifestation of ocular sarcoidosis:

   I. Retinal vasculitis (Periphlebitis) (45-73%)

   II. Vitritis

3735. MC organ affected by sarcoid granuloma in orbit: Lacrimal Gland

3736. MC conjunctival lesion in sarcoidosis: Granuloma

3737. MC location of conjunctival granuloma in sarcoidosis: Inferior palpebral conjunctiva and fornix

3738. MC location of orbital sarcoidosis: Lacrimal fossa

3739. MC fundus finding in sarcoid posterior uveitis: Periphlebitis

3740. MC corneal manifestation of sarcoidosis: Calcific band keratopathy

3741. MC cause of ocular hypertension in sarcoidosis: Nodular infiltration of the trabecular meshwork

3742. MC patterns of sarcoidosis found on ICG angiography:
   I. Hypofluorescent dark spots in the early and intermediate phases of the angiogram which either become isofluorescent or remain hypofluorescent in the late phases.
   II. Focal hyperfluorescent spots seen in the intermediate and late phases
   III. Fuzzy choroidal vessels due to perivascular choroidal leakage in the intermediate phase
   IV. Diffuse zonal hyperfluorescence representing choroidal staining in the late phase of the angiogram

3743. MC neuroimaging abnormalities in sarcoidosis: Meningeal and leptomeningeal enhancing lesions

3744. MC inflammatory etiology of infiltrative optic neuropathies: Sarcoidosis

3745. MC neuro-ophthalmologic manifestation of sarcoidosis: Optic nerve dysfunction

3746. MC orbital manifestation of sarcoidosis: Chronic dacryoadenitis

3747. MC type of vascular occlusion seen in sarcoidosis: BRVO

3748. MC source of a diagnostic biopsy in sarcoidosis: Mediastinal lymph node plexus retrieved by mediastinoscopy

Syphilis

3749. MC presentation of syphilis in eye: Uveitis

3750. MC type of posterior segment involvement of syphilis: Chorioretinitis

3751. MC used nonspecific tests for syphilis:

    I.   Rapid Plasma Regain (RPR) Test

    II.   Venereal Disease Research Laboratory (VDRL) Test

3752. MC used specific test for syphilis:

    I.   FTA-abs (fluorescent treponemal antibody absorbed)

    II.   TPPA (T. pallidum particle agglutination)

3753. MC manifestation of syphilis in HIV positive individuals: Iritis

3754. MC lesion present in an secondary syphilis: Iritis

3755. MC orbital finding in tertiary syphilis: Diffuse bilateral periostitis

3756. MC corneal finding in tertiary syphilis: Uniocular interstitial keratitis

3757. MC bony abnormality in syphilis: Sabre shin on one or both legs

3758. MC CSF abnormalities of neurosyphilis: Leucocytosis (≥5 monBnuclear cells/mm3) and elevated protein (>40 mg/dL)

3759. MC ocular finding of early congenital syphilis: Uveitis

3760. MC ocular finding of late congenital syphilis: Interstitial keratitis

3761. MC intraocular bacterial infection in HIV-positive patients: Ocular syphilis (2% of patients)

3762. MC bacterial cause of Interstitial Keratitis: Syphilis

3763. MC type of syphilis in which Interstitial keratitis occur: Congenital syphilis (90%)

Lyme Disease

3764. MC tick-borne illness in the United States: Lyme disease (LD)

3765. MC ocular finding in early Lyme disease:

   I. Follicular conjunctivitis (11% of patients)

   II. Episcleritis

3766. MC stage wise ocular findings in Lyme disease:

   I. Stage I: Follicular conjunctivitis

   II. Stage II: Anterior uveitis

   III. Stage III: Keratitis

3767. MC posterior segment finding in Lyme disease: Intermediate uveitis (typically bilateral)

3768. MC joint involved in Lyme arthritis: Knee joint

3769. MC cardiac manifestation of Lyme borreliosis: AV block of varying degree

3770. MC neuro-ophthalmic manifestation of Lyme borreliosis: Cranial neuropathy and optic nerve involvement

3771. MC cranial neuropathy of Lyme disease: Seventh CN palsy

3772. MC type of uveitis in Lyme disease: Intermediate uveitis

3773. MC used diagnostic test for Lyme disease:

   I.   ELISA

   II. IFA

3774. MC used treatment for Lyme disease: Oral Tetracycline

Cat Scratch Disease

3775. MC cause of chronic regional lymphadenopathy in children and young adults: CSD (Cat Scratch Disease)

3776. MC etiology of the Parinaud oculoglandular syndrome: Cat scratch disease (An infectious process caused by Bartonella henselae)

3777. MC cause of neuroretinitis worldwide: Cat scratch disease (CSD)

3778. MC posterior-segment/neuro-ophthalmic manifestation of cat scratch disease: Decreased vision with swelling of the optic disc and a macular star figure composed of lipid exudate

MOST COMMONS IN OPHTHALMOLOGY

3779. MC complaint in CSD neuroretinitis: Decreased vision

3780. MC cause of residual visual loss in CSD neuroretinitis: Mild optic nerve dysfunction

3781. MC ocular manifestation of CSD: Follicular conjunctivitis

3782. MC cause of unilateral optic disc edema with a macular star (ODEMS): Cat scratch neuroretinitis

Congenital Rubella Syndrome

3783. MC symptom of congenital rubella: Bilateral or unilateral deafness (44%)

3784. MC systems involved in congenital rubella syndrome:

    I.   Ocular disease (78%)

    II.   Sensorineural hearing deficits (66%)

    III.   Psychomotor retardation (62%)

    IV.   Cardiac abnormalities (58%)

    V.   Mental retardation (42%)

3785. MC ocular manifestation of congenital rubella:

    I.   Rubella retinopathy (occurring in 24% of congenital cases)

    II.   Cataracts (Nuclear MC, often eccentric)

3786. MC cause of poor visual acuity in congenital rubella syndrome:

    I.   Cataract

II. Microphthalmia

3787. MC ocular finding in acquired rubella: Conjunctivitis (70% of patients)

3788. MC lymph nodes involved by rubella infection in children: Posterior auricular, posterior cervical, and suboccipital lymph nodes

3789. MC used serological test for congenital rubella: Serum ELISA

3790. MC complication of postnatal rubella infection: Transient arthritis affecting the small and medium-sized joints

Toxoplasmosis

3791. MC protozoon causing eye disease: Toxoplasmosis

3792. MC Infection of Retina: Toxoplasmosis

3793. MC manifestation of congenital toxoplasmosis: Retinochoroiditis

3794. MC ocular sequelae of congenital toxoplasmosis:

    I. Retinochoroidal scarring

    II. Cataracts

    III. Microphthalmia

    IV. Optic atrophy

    V. Strabismus, nystagmus and phthisis bulbi

MOST COMMONS IN OPHTHALMOLOGY

3795. MC manifestation of acquired toxoplasmosis: Asymptomatic Cervical Lymphadenopathy

3796. MC manifestation of toxoplasmosis in AIDS patients: Toxoplasmic encephalitis/ Cerebral toxoplasmosis

3797. MC presenting symptom of Toxoplasmic retinochoroiditis: Decreased vision and floaters

3798. MC cause of visual loss in ocular toxoplasmosis: Macular scarring and vitreous opacities

3799. MC source of toxoplasma infection:
   I. Ingestion of undercooked Toxoplasma cyst-containing meat
   II. Inhalation or ingestion of oocysts

3800. MC lesion seen in patients with active ocular toxoplasmosis: Focal area of active retinitis greater than one disc diameter in size

3801. MC complication of ocular toxoplasmosis: Secondary glaucoma related to the effects of chronic uveitis

3802. MC location of chorioretinal scarring in congenital toxoplasmosis:
   I. Peripheral retinal scars (64%, most common but not classical)
   II. Macular scars (58%, this is classical but not most common)

3803. MC cause of focal necrotizing retinitis in healthy adults: Toxoplasmosis

3804. MC clinical symptoms of active ocular toxoplasmosis: Blurring or loss of vision and floaters

3805. MC drug combination used for ocular toxoplasmosis: Combination of pyrimethamine, sulfadiazine, and corticosteroids

3806. MC cause of non-viral neurologic disease in patients with AIDS: CNS toxoplasmosis

3807. MC serological test used to diagnose toxoplasmosis: Dye test

3808. MC disease simulating necrotizing viral retinopathies: Toxoplasmic retinochoroiditis

Toxocariasis

3809. MC nematode infection affecting the eye in the United States: Toxocariasis

3810. MC type of ocular lesions in toxocariasis:
   I. Posterior retinal granuloma
   II. Chronic endophthalmitis

3811. MC route of infection of toxocariasis: Ingestion of soil contaminated by toxocara larvae

3812. MC finding in enucleated eyes with ocular toxocariasis: Chronic sclerosing vitritis with secondary total retinal detachment

3813. MC causes of vision loss in Toxocariasis: Vitreous inflammation, CME, and tractional retinal detachment

3814. MC entity confused with Toxocara canis endophthalmitis:

   Retinoblastoma

3815. MC echographic findings in ocular toxocariasis:

   I. A solid, highly reflective peripheral mass (in 91% of patients, the lesion was found in the temporal periphery)

   II. Vitreous membranes extending between the posterior pole and the mass

   III. A traction retinal detachment or fold from the posterior pole to the mass

3816. MC cause of toxocariasis: T. canis

3817. MC cause of Diffuse Unilateral Subacute Neuroretinitis (DUSN): Larva of ascaridoid nematodes including Toxocara canis and the dog hookworm Ancylostoma caninum

3818. MC inflammatory disease that simulates retinoblastoma: Ocular toxocariasis

Cysticercosis

3819. MC ocular tapeworm infection: Larva of Taenia solium (Cysticercus cellulosae)

3820. MC parasitic infection affecting nervous system: Cysticercosis

3821. MC site of infection in ocular cysticercosis: Vitreous

3822. MC presentation of orbital cysticercosis: Restriction of ocular motility

3823. MC extraocular muscle involved in orbital cysticercosis: Superior Rectus

3824. MC clinical finding in intraocular cysticercosis: Vitritis

3825. MC source of cysticercosis infection: Ingesting eggs in contaminated food or water

3826. MC cause of acquired epilepsy worldwide: Cysticercosis

3827. MC parasitic disease of the central nervous system: Neurocysticercosis

3828. MC diagnosed form of cysticercosis: Neurocysticercosis

3829. MC intraorbital parasitic infection:
 I. Cysticercosis
 II. Hydatid cyst (Echinococcus granulosus)

3830. MC helminthic ocular infection: Cysticercosis

HIV AIDS

3831. MC ocular manifestation of HIV-AIDS: HIV Retinopathy

MOST COMMONS IN OPHTHALMOLOGY

3832. MC characteristic of HIV retinopathy: Cotton-wool spots

3833. MC opportunistic retinal infection in HIV-AIDS:

   I. CMV retinitis

   II. Toxoplasmic retinochoroiditis

3834. MC intraocular bacterial infection in HIV-positive patients: Ocular syphilis (2% of patients)

CMV Retinitis

3835. MC clinical pattern of CMV retinitis:

   I. Haemorrhagic (Large areas of retinal haemorrhage on a background of whitened, necrotic retina: "crumbled cheese and ketchup" or "pizza pie appearance")

   II. Brush-fire (yellow-white margin of slowly advancing retinitis at the border of atrophic retina)

   III. Granular (focal white granular lesions without associated haemorrhage)

3836. MC symptom of CMV retinitis: Vitreous floaters

3837. MC mode of progression of CMV retinitis: Old lesion spreading at its borders to involve new previously uninfected retina

3838. MC mode of vision loss in CMV retinitis:

    I.   Prior to HAART: Destruction of infected retina leading to absolute scotoma

    II.   After HAART: Retinal Detachment

3839. MC used systemic drug for CMV retinitis:

    I.   Valganciclovir (900 mg twice daily for 2–3 weeks followed by 900 mg once daily)

    II.   Foscarnet

3840. MC ocular adnexal infection in AIDS patients: Molluscum contagiosum

Misc Uveitis

3841. MC involved region of brain in Intraocular-CNS lymphoma: Frontal lobe

3842. MC ocular finding in Lymphocytic choriomeningitis virus infection: Chorioretinal scarring

3843. MC ocular manifestation of West Nile virus infection: Chorioretinitis

3844. MC complication in Recurrent Uveitis: Glaucoma

3845. MC infectious causes that can mimic a Primary Inflammatory Choriocapillaropathies (PICCP):

MOST COMMONS IN OPHTHALMOLOGY

I. Syphilitic chorioretinitis

II. Tuberculous chorioretinitis

Miscellaneous

Most common Race

3846. MC affected race by sickle hemoglobinopathies: African race

3847. MC affected race by Tay-Sachs disease: Ashkenazi Jews

3848. MC affected race by Idiopathic polypoidal choroidal vasculopathy (IPCV): African-American race

3849. MC affected race by Primary Open Angle Glaucoma (POAG): Black race (African Americans) > Whites

3850. MC affected race by Angle-closure glaucoma: Inuit and Asian

3851. MC affected race by Myopia: Asian > Jews > Black

3852. MC affected race by idiopathic epiretinal membranes: Hispanics

3853. MC affected race by uveal melanoma: Whites > Blacks

3854. MC affected race by HLA-B27-related uveitis and the so-called white-dot syndromes or inflammatory chorioretinopathies: Whites

3855. MC affected race by ocular sarcoidosis and systemic lupus erythematosus: Blacks

3856. MC affected race by Behçet's syndrome: Mediterranean, Middle Eastern, and Asian descent

3857. MC affected race by Vogt-Koyanagi-Harada (VKH) syndrome: Asians, Asian Indians, and Native Americans

3858. MC affected race by Oochronosis: Slovakian and Dominic republic

3859. MC affected race by Oculodermal Melanocytosis: Oriental race

MOST COMMONS IN OPHTHALMOLOGY

3860. MC race affected by hyperopia:

    I.   Hispanic

    II.   Native Americans, African Americans, and Pacific Islanders

    III.   Asians and Caucasians (Least affected)

3861. MC race affected by Oguchi disease: Japanese

3862. MC affected race by sarcoidosis: African or Scandinavian descent

3863. MC race affected by Epiblepharon: Asian

Nutrition Related Disorders

3864. MC ocular diseases attributable to nutritional deficiency:

    I.   Xerophthalmia

    II.   Keratomalacia

3865. MC used clinical indicators of vitamin A deficiency:

    I.   Night blindness or Nyctalopia

    II.   Bitot's spots

3866. MC cause of vitamin A deficiency: Inadequate dietary intake

3867. MC location of lesions in Fundus xerophthalmicus: Mid-Peripheral fundus (a mid-peripheral belt of discreet white spots)

3868. MC laboratory test for the assessment of vitamin E status: Plasma α-tocopherol

3869. MC micronutrient deficiency worldwide: Iron deficiency

3870. MC used indicators of niacin status: Measurements of nicotinamide metabolites in the urine such as N1-methyl nicotinamide and N1-methyl-2-pyridone- 5-carboxylamide (2-pyridone)

3871. MC etiology of folate deficiency: Inadequate dietary intake of folate due to generalized malnutrition or poor nutrition associated with alcohol dependence

3872. MC cause of Vitamin B1 deficiency: Chronic alcoholism

3873. MC ocular finding in infantile scurvy: Unilateral proptosis, sometimes associated with eyelid ecchymoses

3874. MC finding among adults with scurvy: Subconjunctival haemorrhage

3875. MC site of subperiosteal haemorrhage in scurvy: Orbital plate of frontal bone (Left eye more than right)

3876. MC cause of vitamin B12 deficiency: Pernicious anemia

3877. MC quadrant involved in conjunctival xerosis due to vitamin A deficiency: Inferonasal

3878. MC cause of optic neuropathy of malnutrition: Deficiency of vitamin B12

3879. MC clinical signs of copper deficiency: Anemia that is unresponsive to iron therapy

MOST COMMONS IN OPHTHALMOLOGY

3880. MC cause of Lipemia Retinalis (salmon-coloured retinal arteries and retinal veins): Hypertriglyceridemia

3881. MC secondary hyperlipidemia associated with lipemia retinalis: Chylomicronemia from uncontrolled DM

3882. MC defect in galactosemia:
   I. Deficiency in galactose-1-phosphate uridyl transferase (Classical galactosemia)
   II. Deficiency in galactokinase

3883. MC intracellular cobalamin metabolism disorder: Cobalamin C deficiency

3884. MC and most active carotenoids found in human plasma:
   I. Carotene (α-carotene, β-carotene, and lycopene)
   II. 40-carbon hydrocarbons
   III. Xanthophylls (aka oxocarotenoids and includes lutein, zeaxanthin, and β-cryptoxanthin)

3885. MC and stable form of carotene found in foods: All-*trans* isomer

3886. MC used indicator of zinc status: Measurement of serum or plasma zinc concentration

Others

3887. MC causes of ocular UV injuries:

    I.   Unprotected exposure to sunlamps

    II.   Arc welding

    III.   Prolonged outdoor exposure to reflected sunlight

3888. MC used data structure for data exchange between electronic medical record (EMR) systems: HL7 (Health Level 7) (EGS Glaucocard Project)

3889. MC type of Sleep disorder:

    I.   Circadian rhythm sleep disorders (CRSD)

    II.   Sleep disordered breathing

    III.   Parasomnia

    IV.   Restless leg syndrome

3890. MC cause of sleep difficulties today: Excessive or inappropriately timed light exposure leading to CRSD

3891. MC leaning disorder: Dyslexia

3892. MC conditions associated with dyslexia:

    I.   Dysgraphia (writing disability)

    II.   Dyscalculia (math disability)

    III.   Dyspraxia (motor skill and coordination difficulties)

MOST COMMONS IN OPHTHALMOLOGY

3893. MC cause of Empty Sella Syndrome: Pseudotumor cerebri

3894. MC psychiatric symptom in patients with Multiple Sclerosis: Depression

3895. MC subtype of Trichinella: Trichinella spiralis

3896. MC immune deficiency in humans: Selective IgA deficiency

3897. MC urea-cycle defect: Ornithine transcarbamylase deficiency

3898. MC cause of irreversible blindness:

   I. Glaucoma

   II. Age related macular degeneration (ARMD)

3899. MC noted ocular findings in acrodermatitis enteropathica:

   I. Blepharitis

   II. Conjunctivitis

   III. Photophobia

3900. MC cause of nosocomial fungal infection: Candida

3901. MC measurement of antibiotic's potency: MIC (Minimum Inhibitory Concentration)

3902. MC enzymopathy of human beings: G-6-PD deficiency (XLR)

3903. MC congenital defect of Glycosylation: Phosphomannomutase-2 deficiency (PMM2-CDG; previously known as carbohydrate-deficient glycoprotein syndrome [CDG])

MOST COMMONS IN OPHTHALMOLOGY

3904. MC porphyria: Porphyria cutanea tarda (PCT)

3905. MC porphyria associated with ocular surface disease: Porphyria cutanea tarda

3906. MC diagnosed chronic blistering disorder: Bullous pemphigoid (BP)

3907. MC serum immunoglobulin:

   I. Ig G (75%)

   II. Ig A (15-20%)

   III. Ig M (5-10%)

3908. MC malignancy in USA: Carcinoma of the skin

3909. MC skin infection in children: Impetigo

3910. MC autoimmune rheumatologic disease:

   I. Rheumatoid arthritis

   II. Sjögren's syndrome (SS)

3911. MC cardiac manifestation of Rheumatoid arthritis: Pericarditis

3912. MC neuropathy seen in Rheumatoid arthritis: Median nerve compression

3913. MC genetic abnormality in human cancers: Mutations and deletions of p53

3914. MC form of EDS (Ehlers Danlos Syndrome): EDS Type 1 (gravis type)

3915. MC and specific extraintestinal presenting manifestation in Whipple's disease: Migratory polyarthralgias

3916. MC systemic vasculitis:
    I.   Childhood: Henoch–Schonlein purpura
    II.   Adults: Giant cell arteritis

3917. MC endocrine disorder an ophthalmologist will encounter:
    I.   Diabetes mellitus
    II.   Hyperthyroidism

3918. MC microvascular complications of diabetes:
    I.   Proliferative diabetic retinopathy (PDR)
    II.   End stage renal disease (ESRD)

3919. MC Endocrine Emergency: Hypoglycemia

3920. MC hereditary scaling disorder: Ichthyosis vulgaris (IV)

3921. MC complication of adult varicella: Pneumonia

3922. MC encountered form of malignancy in the short term in patients who receive systemic immunosuppression: Post transplant lymphoproliferative disease (PTLD)

3923. MC cause of posttransplant lymphoproliferative disease (PTLD): Epstein-Barr virus (EBV)

MOST COMMONS IN OPHTHALMOLOGY

3924. MC finding of Congenital varicella syndrome (CVS): Cutaneous scars

3925. MC fungal cause of laboratory contamination: A.niger

3926. MC parasitic diarrheal diseases in the world today: Giardiasis

3927. MC manifestation of Mucous Membrane Pemphigoid (MMP): Oral lesions

3928. MC oral lesions in Mucous Membrane Pemphigoid: Desquamative gingivitis

3929. MC involved area in relapsing polychondritis (RP): Pinnae of the ears

3930. MC significant extraglandular manifestation of Sjogren Syndrome (SS): Neurologic disease

3931. MC immunologic finding in Sjogren's syndrome: Hypergammaglobulinemia (polyclonal type)

3932. MC cause of wheezing: Bronchial asthma

3933. MC systemic findings in LCAT (Lecithin- cholesterol acyltransferase) deficiency:
    I. Normocytic anemia
    II. Corneal opacities
    III. Renal insufficiency

3934. MC cardiac manifestation of SLE: Pericarditis

MOST COMMONS IN OPHTHALMOLOGY

3935. caused by synovitis of the wrist

3936. MC cause of death in SLE:

    I.   End stage renal involvement

    II.   CNS involvement

3937. MC neurologic manifestation in SLE:

    I.   Psychiatric illness (Organic Brain Syndrome)

    II.   Seizures

3938. MC cranial nerve affected in SLE: Facial nerve

3939. MC form of myelopathy that occurs in patients with SLE: Transverse myelitis

3940. MC type of Phacomatosis (Neuro cutaneous syndromes):

    I.   Neurofibromatosis

    II.   Tuberous sclerosis

    III.   Sturge Weber Syndrome

    IV.   Von Hippel Lindau disease

3941. MC form of neurofibromatosis: Neurofibromatosis type 1 (NF-1) (von Recklinghausen's disease)

3942. MC abnormality detected on MR imaging in patients with NF1: Foci of increased signal on T2-weighted images in

MOST COMMONS IN OPHTHALMOLOGY

   I. Basal ganglia
   II. Internal capsule
   III. Brainstem
   IV. Cerebellum

3943. MC presenting symptom of NF 2: Bilateral hearing loss

3944. MC type of tumor in NF 2: Schwannomas of the CNS

3945. MC cause of dementia in the elderly: Alzheimer's disease (AD)

3946. MC subtype of seronegative spondyloarthropathies [SSA]: Ankylosing spondylitis (AS)

3947. MC used obesity measure: BMI (Body Mass Index)

3948. MC form of economic evaluation in health care: Cost-effectiveness analysis (CEA)

3949. MC form of human prion disease: Sporadic CJD (Creutzfeldt–Jakob disease)

3950. MC neurologic manifestation of sporadic CJD: Rapidly progressive dementia with myoclonic jerks

3951. MC lysosomal storage disease: Gaucher's disease

3952. MC type of Gaucher's disease: Type 1

MOST COMMONS IN OPHTHALMOLOGY

3953. MC white matter degeneration of childhood: Metachromatic leukodystrophy (MLD)

3954. MC form of MLD: Late infantile form

3955. MC cause of endogenous hyperthyroidism: Graves' disease

3956. MC cause of hyperthyroidism in pregnancy: Graves' disease

3957. MC syndrome of transient hyperthyroidism in pregnancy: Transient hyperthyroidism of hyperemesis gravidarum (THHG)

3958. MC cause of Hypothyroidism: Hashimoto thyroiditis

3959. MC antibody found in patients with Hashimoto thyroiditis: Thyroid microsomal antibody

3960. MC type of chronic thyroiditis: Hashimoto thyroiditis

3961. MC used preparation for treatment of Hypothyroidism: Levothyroxine

3962. MC form of thyroid tumor: Papillary carcinoma

3963. MC type of emboli seen in atherosclerotic disease of the aorta/carotid arteries or cardiac disease:
    I.   Cholesterol emboli (Hollenhorst plaques)
    II. Platelet-fibrin emboli
    III. Calcific emboli

3964. MC iatrogenic cause of stroke: Open heart surgery

MOST COMMONS IN OPHTHALMOLOGY

3965. MC identifiable causes of stroke in adults:

   I.   Cardiogenic emboli

   II. Atherosclerotic occlusive disease

3966. MC cause of stroke in children: Heart disease

3967. MC autosomal recessive spinocerebellar ataxias: Friedreich's ataxia (FA)

3968. MC cause of progressive ataxia in early childhood: Ataxia-telangiectasia (Louis-Bar syndrome)

3969. MC cause of cerebral palsy: Periventricular leukomalacia

3970. MC form of gangliosidosis: GM2 Type I (Tay–Sachs Disease)

3971. MC form of vascular cognitive impairment: Subcortical vascular cognitive impairment

3972. MC systemic findings associated with Aicardi syndrome:

   I.   Vertebral malformations (fused vertebrae, scoliosis, spina bifida)

   II. Costal malformations (absent ribs, fused or bifurcated ribs)

3973. MC enterococci-associated nosocomial infections:

   I.   Urinary tract infection

   II. Surgical wound infection

III. Bacteremia

3974. MC cause of death in Hunter Syndrome (MPS II): Cardiac disease

3975. MC vasculitis of childhood:

   I. Henoch–Schonlein purpura

   II. Kawasaki disease

3976. MC form of arteriosclerosis: Atherosclerosis

3977. MC medical disorder during pregnancy: Hypertension (6-8% of all pregnant women)

3978. MC used scales for accessing level of sedation:

   I. Modified Wilson sedation scale

   II. Observer's Assessment of Alertness/Sedation Scale (OAA/S)

3979. MC pattern of smile:

   I. Mona Lisa smile (67%)

   II. Gummy smile/ canine smile (35%)

   III. Full denture smile (2%)

3980. MC congenital facial anomaly:

   I. Cleft lip and palate

   II. Hemifacial or craniofacial macrosomia

3981. MC associated condition with acute hypertension:

MOST COMMONS IN OPHTHALMOLOGY

    I.   Preeclampsia/eclampsia

    II.   Phaeochromocytoma

3982. MC type of cutaneous T-cell lymphoma:

    I.   Mycosis fungoides

    II.   Primary cutaneous anaplastic large cell lymphoma (CALCL)

3983. MC cause of disability in elderly:

    I.   Arthritis

    II.   Visual impairment

3984. MC cause of cerebrovascular accident (CVA): By embolism or thrombus from an atherosclerotic carotid vessel

3985. MC cerebral artery affected by Internal carotid emboli: Middle cerebral artery

3986. MC life-limiting autosomal recessive disorder among humans: Cystic fibrosis

3987. MC screen reader program for blind users: JAWS for Windows

3988. MC used screen magnifier softwares: MAGic and the ZoomText

3989. MC optical character recognition programs:

    I.   ABBYY FineReader

    II.   Nuance Omnipage

MOST COMMONS IN OPHTHALMOLOGY

3990. MC tauopathy: Alzheimer's disease

3991. MC cause of Congenital Heart Disease:

    I.   Down syndrome

    II.   DiGeorge syndrome

3992. MC disease of exocrine pancreas: Cystic fibrosis

3993. MC way of evaluating renal function in diabetic nephropathy: Measurement of the urinary albumin excretion rates

3994. MC cause of Cushing syndrome: Iatrogenic administration of glucocorticoids

3995. MC features of MEN 1 (Multiple endocrine neoplasia 1): Parathyroid, enteropancreatic, and pituitary tumors

3996. MC endocrine abnormality in MEN 1: Hyperparathyroidism

3997. MC affected area by Solar lentigo: Dorsum of the hands and the forehead

3998. MC factor contributing to resistant hypertension: Excess sodium intake and volume overload

3999. MC used test to measure the effect of heparin therapy: The aPTT (Activated partial thromboplastin time) test

MOST COMMONS IN OPHTHALMOLOGY

4000. MC used test to monitor anticoagulant therapy: The PT (Prothrombin time) test

4001. MC inherited bleeding disorder: Von Willebrand disease (vWD)

4002. MC mosquito-borne viral disease in humans: Dengue fever

4003. MC ocular manifestation of dengue fever: Petechial subconjunctival haemorrhage

4004. MC ocular manifestation of Chikungunya fever: Anterior uveitis and retinitis

4005. MC cause of common cold: Rhinovirus (Picornaviruses group)

www.ingramcontent.com/pod-product-compliance
Lightning Source LLC
Chambersburg PA
CBHW031918240526
45464CB00021B/4